THE DOCTOR GENE

THE DOCTOR GENE

WHAT EVERYONE MUST KNOW ABOUT DOCTORS

DR. RAJAS DESHPANDE

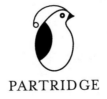

PARTRIDGE

Print information available on the last page.

To order additional copies of this book, contact
Partridge India
000 800 10062 62
orders.india@partridgepublishing.com

www.partridgepublishing.com/india

To
my patients, teachers, students, and friends,
every doctor, nurse, and paramedic upon earth:
thank you.

To
my parents, Dr Kalidas and Dr Usha Deshpande;
my children, Yash and Saarth;
Mrs Tanuja and Mr Abhijit Patki, Shweta, and Shreya;
I am blessed through you all.

Rajas

CONTENTS

SECTION I
THE PATIENT

SECTION II
THE DOCTOR

SECTION III
THE PRACTICE

DISCLAIMER

References to patient's names, locations, and in some cases, events narrated have been changed so as to guard privacy of patients or other individuals. Most of the incidences happened just as described, but I have had to make necessary changes to some events to avoid tracing identities.

True names of some doctors, teachers, colleagues, and some friends appear where relevant, a part of general knowledge.

I smoked cigarettes when I was a student to keep up late nights and quit when I qualified, realizing that it was a mistake. This reference is mentioned where relevant, but I do not support this habit. Smoking is a bad addiction and is by no means to be encouraged.

In case something I have written offends someone for any reason, I apologise in advance and beg forgiveness, also stating that this is not intentional.

Some of my personal opinions, especially in the third section, may not be applicable to everyone. I am open to growth and correction, as every doctor must be.

This is my small prayer for my proud profession.

BEFORE WE MEET

It is indeed a proud joy, being a practising doctor, for there is no more rewarding life than to be able to intellectually solve problems and help people smile again.

There are too many things that go into the making of a doctor, each adding a rich flavour of its own but also enhancing the entire mixture. Sometimes you meet a ripe and sweet part of this mixture, sometimes pickled and sour.

I studied my medical school in India, graduating from a huge set-up with a large number of patients and good teachers but only basic healthcare facilities. It was essential to be able to diagnose based upon 'medical mind chess', deeply thinking about everything to conclude correctly, in the absence of many tests, CT scans, MRI, etc., which are available widely now. Happy that the new technologies have eased life, I feel that it still was an advantage to learn without them. Like the use of a calculator replacing the ready calculations one had in mind as a part of a learning process. A doctor with best of the set-ups in the world, where all technology is state of the art, is still quite inadequate (maybe dangerous) without this clinical training over many years that includes personal interactions with patients and teachers, self-criticism, a massive basic knowledge base, and the ability to handle hundreds of different life-and-death situations while simultaneously dealing with people who are not as educated and sometimes even malicious, angry, and overexpectant.

From the remote farmlands, where I was the only medical care and the nearest medical shop was miles away, to the final referral centres in India or Canada, where the best of the super-specialty education is imparted, all the academic ascent was based upon tough competition at all levels. At all these levels, I met medical angels: teachers and patients who made generations of good doctors. They were also the guardians of all the good principles in medical practice: ethics, morals, extreme hard work and study, best-for-the-patient decision-making, and above all, sacrifices at all levels that are expected of a doctor. This meant personal, social, financial, and mental sacrifices.

India, like most of the developing world, is medically not only backward but also primitive. Except in a few urban pockets, most of the rural population (68 per cent) in India is deprived of good healthcare. In absence of basic infrastructure like roads, transport, electricity, water, sanitation, schools, entertainment, security, and Internet in most of this rural India, the administration expects a well-qualified young doctor to practise there without any equipment, medicine, or support staff. That too at a basic minimum salary lesser than a fourth of what that doctor would earn if he practised in an urban region. There are no financial aids if a doctor wants to make his own set-up in the rural areas.

Medical insurance is not universal, and most of the patients must pay for all their medical expenses. As the cost of living increases, that of investment and equipment flares up, but the poverty-struck society keeps on expecting the doctor to provide the best possible healthcare in a decades-old payment structure. It is unnatural to expect the best talents in the region to practise for charity, capping their income via various laws and rules. There is no mechanism by which the doctor can recover charges from a patient who refuses to pay. It is common to see relatives 'dumping' serious patients in private hospitals and disappearing/refusing to pay. No wonder the helpless doctor is left with two options for a good life: commission-based incomes or emigration to a developed country. Most have chosen the second option. Many who haven't chosen either option are in a perpetual state of financial frustration.

There is no justification of any corruption in any field, including medicine, but there is also no justification for lifelong exploitation of doctors through such one-way laws.

While the society is mostly illiterate and superstitious, the judiciary is yet to awaken to the reality, too busy at present emulating the Western populist medical negligence and ethics judgements to notice the blatant reign of disease, death, lack of medical infrastructure, and the plight of this entire underpaid profession. There is no sorrow like a judiciary that lacks depth of knowledge and the ability to see the big picture. Populist judgments are the newest fashion. There are no examples of judgments reminding/penalizing the government for failure of sanitation and provision of basic healthcare infrastructure. There are no judgments about blatant defamation of the doctors by media.

Almost everywhere in the world now, millions of patients are suffering just because their doctors are making a choice that they can justify to the judicial system rather than what would be their best choice for those patients. It is just to expect to follow laws in a predictable science, but one must know that the human body is extremely complicated and unpredictable. Every doctor in the world now practises under the threat of a litigation.

There is still beauty and hope amidst all this. Many patients speak of their faith and reward their doctors with blessings and prayers, and irrespective of what a doctor earns, the joy of saving lives and treating illness is above any other material achievement. The hidden respect that the majority of society harbours for the medical practitioner is sometimes unleashed as a pleasant surprise in many social events and interactions.

I will never complain about the newer generations being less responsible, as rebellion and revolt are hallmarks of the young, and each successive generation is better equipped with faster and better resources, including their own brains. I am very hopeful that we will achieve good healthcare for everyone in the world in a few years, given the technology we have. However, the new doctors need many infusions about the ways to handle different people, understand and love them, and immense mental strength to resolve the situation rather than submit to it.

My dream is a world where all the doctors in all countries work as one autonomous merit-based organization, using technology to reach out to each individual upon earth to provide the best of medical care. There should be no scope for interference by local laws, political systems, governments, or other organisations. There, of course, must be medical courts to control negligence and other medicolegal issues. There should be wise distribution of funds in research based upon what causes maximum deaths or disability. Everyone should be covered with complete health insurance, and every doctor should be paid according to their skill, time, experience, and complications of a case.

With due respect to all involved, I have always failed to understand the need to spend billions to explore outer space for curiosity, while people here and now upon earth are dying of disease, hunger, and religious violence. Also the wars about boundaries between countries. What do we have to offer to a newfound civilization in space or to the land won by war? Poverty, hunger, wars, diseases that we cannot treat yet, obesity, HIV, beautiful animals on the verge of extinction, global warming, depleting fuel reserves? Many of our existing problems need solutions first. Thinkers are aplenty; vision among the rulers is deficient. We cannot stop infighting between our own people. We cannot unite as a planetary human civilization. What is our stand on unknown species we will encounter? Will we beg for fuel, food, intellect, or wisdom? Our society is sadly often blinded by temporary, meaningless glamour and glitter of an individual or of scientific pursuits and impotent hopes of a better future.

On the famous lists of billionaires and the beautiful, I dream to see doctors, thinkers, philosophers, scientists, environment conservation activists, and humanitarians too, for they are the real beauty of our civilization.

We desperately need more of good, compassionate, hard-working, and intelligent supermen/superwomen called doctors. We all wish for a disease-free world.

This effort is towards that aim.

Thank you, God.

Thank you, Partridge Publishing, Advocate Shrirang Choudhary, Dr Anand and Dr Uma Alurkar, Dr Deepa Muzumdar, Dr Sujata Malik, Mrs Manisha Sanghavi, Dr Susan Zachariah, Dr Joshita Singh, Dr Muthuramalingam Natarajan, Dr Sanjay Singh, Dr Dinesh Kabra, Dr Anka Arora, Dr Sachin Tapasvi, Dr Mrutyunjay Mahindrakar, Dr Nitin Pai, Dr Ketaki Bhonsle-Dhumal, Dr Mudra Parikh, Mr Santosh Kashikar, Mr Bapuguru Vaidya, Dr Malati and Dr Sridhar Vakil, Mr Arvind Deshpande, Dr Kiran Kudrimoti, Mr Rajesh Wattamwar, Dr Aditya Kunte, Dr Chandrima Chuckerbutty, Dr Chetan Puram, Dr Sachin Shah, Dr Sagar Oak, Dr Nilesh, Dr Vinil and Mr Rahil Shah, Dr Anjali and Mr Rajendra Manerikar, Mr Mahavir Shah, Dr Abhay and Dr Jayashree Pohekar, Dr Gajanan Bhalerao, Dr Prachi Jajoo, Dr Meenakshi Kadam, Dr Akshay Oswal, Dr Akshay Jadhav, and my Facebook audience, who have all made my life beautiful.

Special thanks to my colleagues at the Ruby Hall Clinic: Mr Bomi Bhote, Dr Purvez Grant, Dr Ravi Gulati, Dr Bankim Amin, Dr Ashok Bhanage, Dr Sanjay Vhora, Dr Prachee Sathe, Dr Nita Munshi, Dr Jagdish Hiremath, Dr Shirish Hiremath, Dr. Ravindra and Dr Anita Kiwalkar, Dr Lehnaz Umrigar, Dr Venkatramani, Dr Abhay Mutha, Dr Vijay Ramanan, Dr G. Rajasekhar, Dr Sudheer Rai, Dr Srikanta Mohapatra, Dr Sanjay Pathare, Dr Sandeep Karmarkar, Dr Rajesh Parasnis, Dr Surabhi Date, Dr Avinash Nanivadekar,

Dr Rahoul Nagdda, Dr Ashish Atre, Dr Ashish Davalbhakta, Dr Kiran Kharat, Dr Murarji Ghadge, Dr Sheetal Mahajani, Dr Santosh Bhide, Dr Gauri Belsare, Dr Abhijit Lodha, Dr Sanjay Sagar, Dr Sanjeev Tandale, Dr Sachin Arbhi, Dr Vikrant Vaze, Dr Prashant Dev, Mr Sachin Shah (Kalyani Medicals), Mr Manohar Bhosale, Mrs Poonam Chohan, Mrs Nilofer Shaikh, Mrs Anita, all consultants, poly OPD, NTU, ICU, nursing, neurophysiology, parking, cafeteria and security staff, and Mr Pankaj Gaikwad.

Lastly, I think that 'health for all' will be possible if we unite all the healthcare resources globally, prioritise healthcare, and improve the doctor-patient relationship. Utopia was never meant for the weak or the mediocre.

Dr Rajas Deshpande

SECTION I

THE PATIENT

CHAPTER 1

THE REDEEMED DEVIL

Just as I inserted the needle in a patient's spine to obtain the cerebrospinal fluid (brain water), I heard a cacophonic commotion at the ward entrance. The CSF started flowing out drop by drop. A man rushed towards me with a stick in his hand. The ward attendant (an old lady) and a nursing student tried to stop him, but he was too drunk to stop. It was 1 a.m.

It is a delicate procedure and dangerous if the needle hits wrong places like nerve roots or arteries. I could not afford to be physically disturbed at that moment. The assisting nursing student, Ms Reva, fortunately enthusiastic and interested in the procedure, was ready with gloves. I positioned the needle and asked her to hold it, with the sample collection bottle catching the fluid.

I received the first blow upon my shoulder just as I got up from the chair. I asked the second nursing student to help the one holding the needle. I received two more blows upon my back. It was going to take about two more minutes to collect the sample. He slapped me, as I stumbled to avoid falling upon the patient in procedure. I shouted at the ward assistant old lady to call security and engaged with my attacker, trying to restrain him. 'Collect ten ml CSF then withdraw needle with the stylet inside it,' I told the sister (nurse).

This attacker was a stout man in his fifties. His wife had been admitted a week ago in my ward, almost dying. Skin and bones, multiple bedsores and skin infections, stiff all over, high-grade fever, low BP, unconscious. There were curious marks on both wrists and legs, with multiple scars all over her body.

Her husband (my attacker) had admitted her, saying that she was suffering some unknown illness for many months, probably tuberculosis, and had refused to eat. He also told she was a psychotic, under medicines. He offensively smelt of cheap alcohol and lies. He couldn't care less. He disappeared after her admission in the general ward (there was no ICU at our medical college hospital).

A CT scan showed bleeding between skull and brain, with a small fracture over the skull.

Nobody attended her next three days, except her twelve-year-old son who religiously sat crumpled mentally and physically near her. He didn't say anything.

We have an unwritten rule in medicine: the doctor is the caretaker/relative of those who don't have anyone. A true doctor never abandons a helpless patient. Anywhere in the world. It is not taught; it is the basic gene of anyone who is a doctor by heart. We requested our dean (Dr V. L. Deshpande) for a special indent of some high-end antibiotics and other medicines, which he sanctioned. My resident doctor colleagues, Dr Madhu Paulose and others, collected funds to arrange tubes/catheters for her, which were not available in the ward.

On the third day, she opened eyes and reached out to her son's head, patting him. Smiling, she lapsed into sleep again. Even in that sleep, tears rolled down from her eyes, wetting the pillow on both sides of her face.

At the end of that night, around 4 a.m., the child came to me as I sat on the stairs outside the ward, enjoying my customary stimulation that marked the end of the day.

'I want to tell you something,' he said, 'but I am scared.'

I extinguished the stimulant, threw it away.

'Please tell me,' I said, arm around his shoulder. 'Don't be scared. I am with you. I will ensure that all is well.'

'Don't say anything to my father about this. He will throw me out of the house,' he said with a frightened face. I assured him so.

'My father has kept my mom in the basement room of our house for many years now. He ties her hands and legs and even her mouth every day. I go down and give her food and water two times a day. He allows me that but tells me that I should not tell anyone about it. There is a small bathroom in the basement, which she can use, but if tied, she soils her clothes and then cleans

4

up next time I untie her. Our relatives are all scared of my father—he is violent often. He even has friends among the police. He drinks alcohol every day. We earn some money from the rent of another apartment. Both the houses belong to my mother. If someone asks about her, we tell she is sick and the doctor has not allowed her to meet anyone. If she cries or shouts, Papa beats her up with fists, kicks, or a stick. She has been having fever since more than a week. Papa thought she will die now. So he shifted her here. Will she survive?'

I was all trembling, young and boiling blood. 'We are trying our best, friend,' I told him and asked, 'Do you have any other relative who can help you?'

'I have an aunt who stays in another town. My father told her that he will kill my mother if she interferes, so she doesn't.'

'Please ask her to come over. Call her today. I will ask our operator to connect,' I told him.

The next morning, I reported this in confidence to our dynamic RMO, Dr Annasaheb Mhaske. He arranged for the local police in hospital to enquire about the case with her relatives and neighbours. The patient's sister came over, and the kid was sent with her.

Hence this attack. As I tried to dodge his blows, the drunk husband started abusing. I requested that we fight out of the ward; he could beat me there. He suddenly pushed me and ran to the bed where his wife, a face of fear, now conscious, was looking at us. We all lost patience with him and actually grabbed him, knocking him over, dragging him out of the ward as he made a fracas. The two constables on duty had rushed to the ward; they took him over with two justified slaps and left the ward.

The student sister had withdrawn the needle after collecting the sample, waiting for me to seal the pierced point. I washed hands, put on gloves, and sealed it.

The police station called for me. Dr Mhaske, our RMO, waited there. The violent attacker was tied down (restrained) to a chair. Dr Mhaske asked if I wanted to file a complaint against him for attacking me (this was the period before any laws for attacking hospital staff/doctors were made). I declined.

In a surprise move, the police constable, who was quite upset that this drunk had attacked a ward doctor, asked me to slap or kick him if I wanted, now that he was tied down.

I didn't want to, but I was seething with the anger of his interference in my procedure risking someone's life. I went to him and held his shirt collar, wanting to thrash him verbally.

I looked at him.

'Bloodshot eyes, distended veins upon the face, pulsatile neck vessels, sweating, breathlessness . . .' Could he be developing a heart attack, high blood pressure? I requested Dr Mhaske that he be taken to the casualty. He agreed. His BP was very high, and the ECG showed a strain pattern. He was admitted and treated, improved.

His wife refused to launch a complaint against him. He promised the police and wife's relatives to treat her fair. We arranged for his counselling for quitting alcohol and other issues.

The kid came a few months later with his mom to the ward. She was near normal; both were smiling. 'Today is my son's birthday, Doctor,' said his mother. 'We wanted to give you and your ward staff these sweets.'

The happy nursing staff gathered around her.

I gave him the fountain pen I had in my pocket as a birthday present.

I was just a poor resident doctor.

'We went to the Ganesh temple this morning to pray for you,' said the kid to me.

I was also the richest.

CHAPTER 2

A MOTHER WHO
KILLED THE WIFE

'He is angry with us, Doctor. He refuses to recognise me, even his parents and children sometimes. It was all my fault. I fought with him so many times over small things. I have said sorry so many times now. But he is not ready to talk again like he did. Some doctors said he is in shock. Some advised psychiatric treatment. We did all we were told, but he is worse by the day. Please bring him back, Doctor!' said the extremely depressed and tearful middle-aged lady. On her lap was a five-year-old daughter; seated behind her were her in-laws (patient's parents) and her elder child, a nine-year-old boy. My professor was listening carefully, and we neurology residents were juggling possibilities in our minds.

I was assigned the workup of this case. After a week-long evaluation and opinions of some senior neurologists in Mumbai, it was concluded that he was an exceptional case of early-onset Alzheimer's disease. The patient, Mr Bhooshan, an electrical engineer, was about thirty-nine years old then.

Every morning that I entered the ward, I found his wife begging him to forgive her and talk normally again. He looked at her blankly, often irritated and with a questioning face. She would bring the kids to him every evening and prod them to talk to him, crack jokes, and in general, 'get him to talk'. He would occasionally call them near himself, pat them, then suddenly vanish mentally from the scene. He sometimes asked his wife about them by names but didn't always recall the names accurately. Somehow, children sense moods excellently. They tend to know when a parent is disinterested or 'just not there'. These kids did whatever their mother suggested, but they were okay with just sitting by his side, in his lap, holding his hand.

I never saw his aging parents without teary eyes that begged for relief from this hell.

We have different memory areas in brain for sights, smells, words, etc., as well as disciplined cascades of time-based memories. A large part of this is what we call the past. Hidden therein is also our knowledge of ourselves: name, birth, family, culture, religion, education, friends, nature, everything that makes someone's personality unique to them.

Imagine losing parts of this memory, references to yourself. Imagine not knowing who you are. Imagine being lost inside your own mind. Then also imagine not even knowing that you are lost. It is only initially that the patient knows and cares about such loss of memory. Unlike dramatic depictions of violent anger because of forgetting things in some movies, patients usually also lose their concern/insight about what is happening to them.

There is a point of no return in the mental/cognitive decline in patients with dementia/memory loss, comparable only to the death of one's mind as one knows it. Scary.

Relevant medicines were started. There was a negligible response.

Mr Bhooshan gradually became almost blank and spent most of his day in the bed, often wandering aimlessly and watching windows in the ward. His wife couldn't come to terms with this. She mostly just sat in a corner, often crying whenever kids visited. Right from prayers to herbals, everything that anyone suggested was being done by the family.

Our counsellors talked to her, even prescribed for her mild antidepressants, but she had just collapsed inside.

One evening, I didn't see her by the patient. Curious, I enquired about her to the patient's mom who was instead attending him. 'Their daughter, the five-year-old, is admitted in the paediatric ward below with high-grade fever. She is with her,' replied the old lady.

I went to the paediatric ward after finishing my duty.

I found the kid in bed, weak but comfortable and smiling. Her mother, the patient's wife, was telling her funny stories, laughing aloud and imitating comical characters as she fed the child. Mrs Bhooshan was a totally different lady then. She talked to me very nicely, without any hint of hiding sorrow naturally. The innocent, happy kid invited me to sit by her and share her food.

In two days, the kid was discharged. Her mom had completely changed. She started taking good care of Mr Bhooshan again, but now with a mysterious peace upon her face, often smiling and mothering her husband too, like her other kids.

Satisfied with the sacrifice that this mother had made by killing the wife within herself, life had smiled upon them again in the face of an obvious tragedy. They returned home, and she was still nursing him and looking after the kids one year later when I passed my exams and left Mumbai.

Their life had changed but moved on.

So had mine. I started writing a diary.

CHAPTER 3

THE SUICIDE NOTE
OF A DOCTOR

'Insecticide poisoning. Needs intubation. Quick!' I shouted and started suction from the frothing mouth of this twenty-seven-year-old Ayurvedic practitioner. The casualty servant rushed the primitive version of a crash cart that had the bare minimum upon it and relied upon the cosmic arrangement of a maximum of two emergencies at a time and enough time between the second and third to wash and sterilise the instruments.

Positioning his neck in extension, I realised that there was no light in the laryngoscope. The nurse knew this, so she automatically held a torchlight, and I could aspirate the bloodstained froth. The glass bottle of the manual suction pump, where the ward boy had to pump it to generate negative pressure, started filling fast.

'Doctor, his pulse is forty,' said the young lady standing by his side. Calm face, tremulous, heavy voice. Red eyes watering without knowing it. Distracting. I saw the vocal cords and inserted the tube. The ward boy had kept the ambu bag (artificial respiration rubber bag) ready. We started the routine medicines to increase pulse rate and reverse the respiratory paralysis.

There were no ventilators or ICU. No ABG analysers or pulse oximeters.

'I am his wife,' said the graceful lady. 'We both practise in this village near Nanded, started a year ago. Six months ago, he was diagnosed with bone cancer with multiple secondaries. One month ago, he had become paralysed because of a spinal secondary. He doesn't want to live any more. Today, he crawled in to our farm behind our house and took this poison' she said.

He stabilised by morning. She didn't leave his side at all. They took turns: sisters, ward boys, his parents, and her, with the ambu bag. The next day, he started breathing on his own. He pulled out the tracheal tube himself and, fortunately, maintained his respiration.

Having just passed MBBS and in my internship, I was too junior to counsel him. So I decided to just tell him how much his wife had exerted to save his life. That would probably help his depression, I thought.

I told him so. He said he wanted to talk to me when she was not around. That evening when she went home to change, I went to the doctor-patient.

'Please help me. Please understand, my friend . . . you are too young to understand, but please try,' he said to me, after I assured him that our discussion will be confidential. 'My wife is pregnant, two months. I want her to abort. You see, I won't probably even live to see the baby. Who doesn't want their baby? But if she becomes a mother, she will never get to marry a good match again. She is so beautiful and intelligent. I love her. Let her start a new life after me. If she delivers this child, she will always keep thinking about me. You see, she loves me so much that she wants to have the child just as my memory after me. She does not want to marry again. Will you let that happen to someone you love? If I die now, she will still have some time to abort. My father will convince her, and she may change her mind if I am not around. Let me go, please.'

God helped me in that dilemma. He improved well and was discharged. I could barely look into his eyes. I was bewildered with this situation.

Within a week, a colleague who knew him told me that the young doctor had died, bleeding himself to death, cutting his own wrist. I asked if I could meet his wife. I wanted to tell her how much he cared for her. He passed on the message.

The bereaved young lady doctor came over after a month. We had tea in the casualty. I told her what had happened, just because I didn't want her to blame him for killing himself. Also, she had the right to that information, now that he was no more.

'I know, Doctor. Thank you. He wrote me a note before dying. He also mentioned that he had talked to you. I am okay now.'

I was extremely curious about her decision about her pregnancy but could not bring myself to ask her about it. She was about my age. 'Somehow I feel responsible for you like a brother, because he confided in me. Please let me know if you ever need anything. I will do my best,' I told her.

'I will start my practice in a different place, Doc, where I can forget him. That was his last wish—that I marry again and forget him. He also wanted me to abort—he wrote so in the note. So I did.' She looked away to hide tears.

I realised I was tearful too and didn't know what to say.

Suddenly, there was a rush and panic, and in came a frothing patient.

She waited patiently till I stabilised the new patient, handed over to a colleague, and calmed down the relatives.

'Bye for now,' she said with a weak smile as she left.

Then, turning back, she pulled a neatly folded paper, a photocopy of his last note, and held her finger at this:

> I will not watch you from the heaven or the sky. Please find
> love once more.

CHAPTER 4

HUMANS?

Two a.m., about twenty years ago. Casualty, civil hospital, Nanded. World asleep.

In came rushing a crowded jeep. Panicked passengers carried someone in a blood-soaked bed sheet. Huge bearded man in forties. Heavy bodybuilder. White kurta pyjama (dress) now blood red. Hacked by many with machetes (kukri), swords, knives.

From head to toe, innumerable cuts. Breathing fast, shallow. Eyes open, looking at us whenever fluctuating consciousness allowed. They had an expression without pleading or pain. He knew what was coming. Probably a combination of hope and gratefulness. He couldn't talk.

He was a sarpanch (political head) of a nearby village, a known criminal, rapist, and murderer and was thus punished by the villagers whom he had offended. His cousin accompanying him told us. Remaining people left as fast as they came. In a patient cut at over a hundred places but still alive, where does one start? No ICU. OT not functional. Nearest big city Hyderabad, eight hours away. No blood donors. Blood sent for grouping; transfusion started. We ran around, but the inevitable kept torturing us all its life. In about twenty minutes, he died.

Those eyes with an expression I can't name lived on in my mind.

* * *

A known gangster, age nineteen, was admitted critical, stabbed by a rival gang leader. They had had a fight over a girl. The murder was planned months ahead; the knife used was said to have been coated with some chemical/herb known to be a sure-shot killer. The threat of this planned murder had already circulated in some groups. His statement was recorded by police.

As I started the blood transfusion (an intern's job), awaiting him to be shifted for emergency surgery, he whispered to me, barely managing these words: 'Please save me, Doctor. That girl was mine. I must kill him. Please save me. I will give you anything you want. But I want to kill him.'

'Calm down. Take a slow, deep breath. We will try our best. We have started the medicines—you'll be okay.' I reassured him, best I could.

He held my hand and squeezed it. 'I love her, Doctor. Save me. I cannot die with this feeling. She was mine. I want to take revenge.'

The poison worked early. He sank even before he could be shifted to the OT.

His last words of revenge lived on in my mind.

* * *

'What do you do?' asked my lecturer to this shackled prisoner in the infectious ward, admitted for cholera. Scars were his face.

'I am a sharpshooter. Supari murderer [contract killer].' He was in his twenties. He had no expression upon his face.

I was always idealistic. He was my age. Late that night, after all work, I went to him. He was sitting blankly with his guard from prison, who read a newspaper.

'Where are your parents?' I asked this patient.

After a pause, he answered, 'My father was also in this line. He's dead. I took revenge for him then started this job.'

'And your mother?'

'Why do you ask all this? When will I be discharged?'

'In two days,' I answered, and asked again pleadingly. Somehow I was curious about his mother.

'She killed my father to run away with her lover. I killed that lover. She is in another jail.'

There still was no expression on his face.

'Can I smoke a cigarette?' he asked me.

14

'Not here,' I told him and winked at the guard, who took out his bidi (country cigarette) bundle.

I offered him hospital tea and just sat there.

He appeared a bit relaxed. 'I have a little sister in my state, twelve years old, in a boarding school. I want her to become a doctor like you'.

'She will,' I said, happy, not knowing why! 'I am sure you will help her.'

It was then that he looked at the sky and smiled a smile that tore through chains of shame, guilt, agony, and helplessness.

'It was her birthday yesterday,' he said and then he looked at me.

That face again had no expression, but it made burning scars upon my mind.

CHAPTER 5

HOMICIDE OF A PATIENT

Tuesday, 3 p.m., OPD

'She needs urgent admission and treatment . . . she may be developing a stroke.' I told the relatives of this seventy-some-year-old lady who was having recurrent episodes of tingling/numbness all over her body, with slurred speech. Otherwise healthy.

The disturbed family was displeased: a mother (patient), her son, and her daughter (very polished but obviously cut off from each other because they avoided talking to each other), who stayed in different cities away from the patient. 'You can suggest us the treatment and tests, Doctor,' the US-based son said, 'but it is difficult to admit her, as there is no one to stay with her in the hospital. I am in India only for three days, and I reached Pune only yesterday. I am very worried about Mom, so got her here today . . . but I have to return as we have an important project going on that depends entirely upon me.'

'I am not sure if she will agree for hospital admission, Doc' said the daughter. 'She is very independent, never liked hospitals . . . Do you want to stay in the hospital, Mom?' she asked the patient. The question had anxiety, reluctance, formality, and suggestion for a negative answer all at the same time.

The mom looked at me with an embarrassed smile, confused. 'Well, if it is necessary—' she started, only to be cut off by her daughter. 'Let the doctor write the treatment and tests, Ma, then we will decide outside.'

I suggested an urgent MRI and a few other tests and gave a prescription. 'Do we have to do the tests here only, Doc? Because we know that X trust, and its chairman is a very close friend of mine.'

This trust was known for free MRIs, average quality, meant to serve the poor. It takes time to get the appointments there, and some poor patient's appointment would be cancelled because this 'chairman's friend from the US' would request an urgent MRI.

'It is your choice,' I had to answer legally correct, even if I did not like this decision.

I wrote notes, suggested urgent admission, and started treatment.

Four days. No follow-up.

Then on Saturday at 6 p.m., the casualty MO called, 'Sir, you had seen this patient in OPD on Tuesday. She has come here. She is comatose—we are planning to intubate.'

I went there, anguished to the core but trained to shut up well when dealing with patients. The daughter rushed to provide details: 'Doc, she was not willing for admission on that day. We did the MRI at the trust hospital yesterday morning, but she was very sleepy since the prior night. We got the report last evening. We thought she must be tired, so we waited till now, but she is not waking up . . . Then we thought that you advised admission, so we brought her here.'

Patient had had a brainstem stroke, one of the worst forms of stroke.

'When did she become unconscious exactly?' I asked. (This is how the court wants answers, ain't it?) Our intention was to see if she was in the window period for clot-busting treatment of stroke.

'The servant says about two days, but I saw her day before yesterday, and she said she was okay . . . I stay nearby only and am in constant touch with her and the servant on phone.'

There was no point in discussion; they had all explanations about all decisions and why things were delayed.

She required a ventilator. The 'busy' son kept on calling from the United States and had their 'doctor uncle in the US' talk with us, conducting an accented cross-examination on the phone and telling us what we already knew. On the third day, the family gathered all its socio-financio-politico-legal experts of clever talk and asked for a meeting. This discussion ensued, summarily:

'When exactly will she regain consciousness?'

'Can't say.'

'How many more days in the ICU?'

'Can't say.'

'Will she ever talk or walk again?'

'Can't say.'

'Will she be a "vegetable"?'

'Can't say.'

One smarty-pants (well, smarty half-pants) asked with dismay, 'But, Doctor, medical science has made such great advances in the USA. They say stroke patients can be treated completely. They have even done stem cell transplants, etc., and you are saying we can't do anything.'

I knew a hundred hurtfully true answers that could expose the questioner. But again, my teachers shouted in my mind, 'Shut up!'

'At this stage, after the stroke has happened, we cannot do much' was the technical answer.

'Doc, please understand the family's situation—how long can we continue this?'

'What can I do to help?' asked I.

The family exchanged meaningful glances. Smarty half-pants conjured up the big courage. 'We are ready to accept the inevitable. It is okay if you tell us she is not going to survive. We are prepared.'

I offended my teachers once in my mind to answer that one. 'But you all have already killed her by delaying her treatment.' I couldn't say it openly.

They waited another two days.

Then requested not to resuscitate the patient.

Besides the question 'When?' they were not interested in anything else. The more we tried, the more that family started hating us, alleging us, questioning us. If we advised any new medicine, the first question was 'Will it definitely make any difference?'

I will not mention when the family was seen smiling last.

So many patients die/develop disabilities because the family denies them medical care in time. Super-precious time is wasted in second opinions, finding cheaper options to everything, and idiotic presumptions and self-medication. Add to this some alternative medicines that are cheaper and available at home.

Many parents don't ensure the availability of important drugs like epilepsy medications of their own children, do not stock in advance, and take huge risks by trying on their own to stop these medicines.

Many among the elderly population are, to state honestly, 'killed by neglect masked by beautiful, sweet language and excuses'; only few exceptions are seen in real life.

Wives are taken for granted for the treatment of husbands (the earning member) in the family, however serious their health problems may be. Critical/crucial surgeries are avoided; admission advice is neglected because the patient/relatives keep on searching for the cheapest or easiest options.

Patients too sometimes continue to neglect the doctor's instructions—eating sweets, not exercising as advised, drinking alcohol and smoking, driving riskily, quoting 'It's my life.' Then why is the doctor held responsible when one develops complications of such a life?

All these delays cause more deaths than medical negligence by doctors. There must be a law to record and punish these too. Hospitals must also have a registry of admissions advised and investigations suggested, and in case they are not followed, they must report such cases for medical negligence.

Where the court decides the punishment amount for doctor's negligence by calculating how much the dead/disabled person would have earned, what else do we expect? This is like an open legal statement: if a doctor neglects the health of a non-earning or an elderly member or when the parents have many sons, it deserves lesser compensation, but if an earning member/only child is affected by negligence, the hospital/doctor pays up huge! This is a law promoting legal inequality, stating that an earning young human being's life is superior to any other!

As for the smarty half-pants, it will take him just a few more years to understand how his mother felt in the last days of her life.

CHAPTER 6

THIS CRUEL DILEMMA

'You will die soon. You may want to prepare. You have maybe three years left,' said my professor to a patient with CBGD, a grave neurological diagnosis.

The elderly Canadian lady and her daughter broke down, screaming and hugging each other. Weak in such situations, I stood there trembling, trying to control tears. After a coffee and lots of water, the patient reassured her daughter, 'It's OK, dear, the doctor has to see other patients too. Thank you, Doc, for seeing us.' They left with the prescription. Besides being shattered, the daughter was visibly fuming at my professor. I felt offended too by what he had done.

After the OPD, I angrily asked my professor, 'Couldn't you have made it softer? I'm sorry, but I thought that was quite blunt and rude.'

'It's the law. You must tell the truth to the patient. And it is my experience that the lesser the words used, the better it is. They will suffer now but learn quicker to accept it.'

'I disagree, sir. Does law presume that all patients are made up of the same scientific and logical mindset as robots? Some may be very emotional, sensitive, anxious, depressed, and in fact die early with such news. Not everyone wants to know the truth this way. You could have told her about just a suspicion now and confirmed later when she would be better prepared to hear it.'

'Then she would have died every day till I confirmed it. Now she will not,' said the prof. 'And anyway, there's always a question of legal aspects of delaying the news.'

I didn't sleep that night. I have always felt that a patient's life is never the same once a bad diagnosis is confirmed, so unless it is essential to specifically state it (or the patient asks for it) the 'death' part must be excluded from the first discussion (unless urgent/emergent measures are mandatory to prevent it). One cannot hide the truth, but then one should not take for granted a patient's sensitivity or emotional tolerance level.

Back in India.

Here, requests like 'Please don't tell the patient her diagnosis, she is very sensitive' are as common as rude children asking the approximate time to you-know-what in front of the patient.

This twenty-four-year-old lady living alone (fought with family, mom in another city) came with mild weakness in one leg. Examination was suspicious for some brain problem. MRI was advised. She went home after the MRI. I received an email report of her MRI that midnight. Huge tumour, likely cancerous. Restless, I went through a bad night again, angry about why such things happen and worried about how I should tell this to her.

The next day, she came to the OPD.

'Do you have any relative who can come over to discuss?' I asked.

'I had a break-up last week. So none. You can tell me,' she said, plain and dignified.

Fumbling carefully with language, I told her that she had a tumour in the brain and may need operation. I carefully mentioned in passing that it may be cancerous in some patients.

Without a change in her expression, she asked, 'Can we do the surgery tomorrow?'

Stunned, I repeated details of her MRI, now more direct.

'Yes, I understand it might be cancer, I need a surgery, and I can die during the surgery.

I will call my mom. I am ready for admission now,' she said plainly again.

She was operated a day later by a neurosurgeon colleague.

Her mom came over for surgery.

The biopsy was negative for malignancy.

She is now back to life, full swing, and on her last visit showed me the steps of Zumba that she had recently learnt.

I wish I could dance like her. Life too.

I have not met another patient like her yet!

What is the best way to say bad news?

If the doc says it all, they are going to scare and worry themselves to sleepless nights and a disturbed life for a long time, whether literate or not. Professional duties demand that one explains the truth in the best and most compassionate language possible. Knowledge of human nature teaches us that however 'downplayed' you may convey the diagnosis, a patient will think only of the worst (the very reason why doctors themselves make the worst patients). If we don't tell the real risks involved in the progression of that disease, patients will not take it seriously and will continue to risk their lives, not do the advised tests, or neglect the suggested treatment. If we do tell, there is a feeling that the doc is trying to extort via tests, etc. What helps here is the continuous, real-time assessment of the patient's nature and finding the right relative balanced enough to confide in, with the patient's consent. Sometimes in patients who are overtly depressed and are at a suicidal risk, the doctor may have to withhold information (unless immediately life-saving) for a while until a proper occasion.

In the west, there mostly are counselling or meeting rooms and a social worker or counsellor present while gently breaking such news to the patient. Often, in cases of large, irate, or violently oriented patients, there are security personnel guarding the room too. In India, the concept is evolving and more needs to be discussed, considering a large number of excessively emotional, illiterate, and often denial-oriented population, mob mentality, and many prevalent superstitions. People also avail of many FDA-unrecognised alternative therapies even at the cost of their own life.

Many doctors are equally sensitive and emotional, and I have seen colleagues who suffer patients' bad news.

There is no doubt that the patient must be told the truth, but prediction of time of death (unless in emergencies where it is obvious) should be avoided. There are medical miracles. Even some cases of rabies have survived, and some cancers didn't progress as predicted or were cured with treatments. There are cases, like that of Prof. Stephen Hawking, who have (productively) survived far beyond their predicted ALS death.

All said and done, the doctor is not God to predict. Prognosis is a dynamic statistical entity.

The patient's courage matters as much as their morale in their survival. The doctor should guard both. One can only mention statistics in carefully chosen compassionate words. I also find it useful to tell the patient that 'come what may, I am, in this battle, on your side.'

May all patients, doctors, and relatives find their own peace with all the bad news that they must deal with. There are thousands of doctors who die their patients' death. Not everyone can express their agonies. No doctor sleeps well for weeks after a death.

Bad news should not be made worse. Careful words are as important as connecting with the patient mentally.

Death, you see, is never felt by the dead. It is only life that suffers the news of death.

CHAPTER 7

THE TORTURED BELOVED

'I want to kill my father, Doc. Is there any way?' said the polished lady.

Used to a life full of shocks, cruelty, and in general, many negative shades of human behaviour, we learn to mask emotions to avoid turning off the patient /relative from telling us the whole truth.

This was a googly, and I made a conscious effort to retain my composure.

Thirty-something, very posh, and from a high-class, cultured family, this lady was one of those who automatically garner respect of people around them. What she said didn't fit in with the mental image she had impregnated upon my mind. Could she be one of the PSY cases?

'I live with two daughters aged nine and fourteen. My mom passed away ten years ago. My husband stays away as he cannot tolerate my father. My father was a military officer, retired with many honours. About five years ago, he started forgetting things. We took him to many doctors all over. They said he had dementia. Two, three years ago he started abusing in the worst filthy and obscene language we never thought he could use. He also started getting naked anywhere and doesn't care if I, my daughters, or neighbours are around. He passes urine deliberately when in public and around us. He also makes attempts to sexually abuse us all and tried more than once to grope the maids, who then quit. We had a hard time when a maid filed a police complaint. I could not dump him as no one else can look after him. So I nursed him at home, and my husband, who could not tolerate this daily abuse, left us to stay in another state.' She started sobbing.

All I could offer was a few tissues and a coffee. I waited for her to speak again.

'I am sorry,' she said in a wet, guilty, embarrassed, and one of the most pained voices I had heard. 'I love my father as much as I love my husband. I cannot dump my father. But then I cannot let my daughters go through this every day. They are terrified and have started behaving strangely. We took him to many psychiatrists, and they gave medicines that kept him calm, but he developed too many side effects and could not move out of bed. Now he refuses to take any medicines, and if we force him, he gets violent.' Again, amongst sobs, she showed me her swollen, blue-black shoulder.

'I have to tie him up to his bed and lock his room at night, but he keeps shouting. Our neighbours have started asking us to either dump him or move out of the society. The old-age homes here do not accept such patients.'

'I am a personality development counsellor, but my work is suffering now. I have lost my smile. I have lost my life. I cannot die. I have two kids to raise. So I want my father to die. Is there any legal, medical way to kill him?' And then a volcano of unvoiced pain of years wailed out through her throat. She kept her head on the table and cried.

It was unprofessional, but I had to get up and pretend to wash hands just to be able to wipe tears in my own eyes.

Fronto-temporal dementia, a cousin of Alzheimer's dementia, is a condition in which, along with progressive memory loss, there is abnormal behaviour, delusions, sexual inappropriateness, etc. It happens due to degeneration in some parts of the brain. It is progressive for about five to twelve years till the patient develops some fatal complication.

This was not totally new. I remember many patients who are tied up at home, beaten up cruelly by their family, and left to die due to this kind of behaviour. This tragic management is also commonly meted out to many psychiatry patients, who are burnt, injured with sharps, shackled, and tied to beds/trees, kept with head under running water, and even poisoned/sedated with herbal or even allopathic medicines to ensure safety of those around them.

Few years ago, one family of bodybuilders (all three brothers in land business) admitted their father with the complaint 'He burnt himself with hot water in the bathroom.' There were many bruises too. 'He fell at home.' they said. When the sons left, the servant told the resident doc, 'They [patient's sons] threw boiling water upon his genitals after tying and beating him because he tried to grope his eldest daughter-in-law.' This patient had severe Parkinsonian features too, so he was not able to move much due to stiffness. They had beaten him up and burnt him in that condition!

The lady in front of me regained her calm in a few minutes. I explained to her what many neurologists and psychiatrists may have earlier told her many times, about such being the nature of this disease. However, we have many safer medicines to control psychosis now. I wrote her a prescription and promised her that I would try and locate a care centre for such patients with this severe level of psychosis. There were none in that city. The next option was to hire a strong male attendant and rent a small single room apartment nearby where she could shift her father. Her husband shifted back. The family appeared to gradually recover from the bad days.

As much as we need the doctors to explain the family about such illnesses, we also need to educate our society about such conditions and care homes for these patients. Inhuman beating up, tying down, injuring, poisoning, and humiliating fates by one's own children is probably the worst that can happen to a human being.

When the lady came to visit with her daughters few months later, her cute daughters greeted me mannerfully. We, all the grown-ups, avoided the topic of 'sick Grandpa'. However, the nine-year-old, while leaving, boldly asked her mom's permission to ask me a question.

Then looking straight in my eyes, the kid asked me, 'Doc, why did God do this to my Grandpa? Is it possible to cure him? We used to enjoy so much together. I was his dearest. It is okay if he hurts me—I want him back.'

I cursed my stunned wits. 'He will get better soon, dear,' I lied to the cute little one.

CHAPTER 8

THE LAST MEDICINE

'Do you love someone too much, Duck-toor?' asked this Iraqi student in hesitant words with an awkward face. He was just translating what his countryman had insisted him to ask me.

A young lady in her late twenties was paralysed below the neck, and her husband had risked his life to smuggle her out of Iraq. He had dropped his kids at his sister's home in Turkey and flew her to India for treatment. He knew no one here, and one Iraqi student was being a Good Samaritan to the couple.

'Yes,' I replied, with a thousand resounding echoes within my mind.

'My friend here says if you love someone, then only you will understand that if his wife dies, he will not be able to live.' said the interpreter.

'Please tell him I understand.' I said. 'We are trying our best, but he must know that she is critical right now.'

The unfortunate lady, who had been bedridden for weeks at home, had developed a blood clot that had reached her lungs. Her oxygen levels were dropping. She was in the ICU, breathless, and her expression was beyond fear; her eyes cursed her own life.

'He says please try for his wife just like you would try for your beloved. Do not worry about money, he will arrange anything required,' said the translator, hesitant again, knowing that this may be misused.

'Please tell him that money is not the problem at all. The treatment is already on. We must wait for improvement now,' I assured him. I am yet to see a doctor who abandons treatment of a serious patient for money.

The husband, like most Middle Eastern patients, wore a new coat, a mark of respect for a new country, especially when visiting a doctor. Strong-built, resolute-faced—it was a torture to see him break down without any external signs. His eyes never had tears, but his face was a painting of a crying heart. Day in and day out, he sat by his wife, holding her hand, speechless except when she asked him something.

Whenever they looked at each other, my heart knocked the divine door violently.

On the fifth day, she came out of ICU. On the tenth, she was walking with the help of a walker.

The next day when I visited her, the hubby was out for some police work (visa), and she (patient) told the interpreter something for me. For the first time in my life, I saw the interpreter crying. He told me, 'Sir, her husband's parents were killed in the war just a week before this couple came to India. Even this family was trapped. They have three kids. Their elder daughter, aged twelve, saw her neighbour's home bombed and now wakes up often in the night, scared. She is attending the two younger ones, ten- and seven-year-olds, at the home of their relative in Turkey. Her husband sold his shop in Iraq to bring her here. Please give them the best medicines so she can meet her children soon again and take care of her family.'

I am not made up of stone. My poise wavered, and I was fighting tears.

'Please tell her that I will do everything for her as I would for my sister.' I defied the Western medical etiquette: never to patronise. But it is difficult to talk logical, businesslike technicalities to someone who meets you with an open heart. A doctor, however much skilled, unless also first a human being, appears like an emotionless wax statue to the patient.

She smiled and showed me an old picture of hers with her three sweet kids.

I requested my boss, and he agreed for billing concessions too. But the patient's husband declined to accept the concession. He told the translator, 'A deal is a deal. We must pay, and he must accept.' Finally, he forced me to accept a token dinar as their memory. Fond of the fantasy of the *Arabian Nights*, the word *dinar* still carries an alluring aura in my mind.

On the day that they left, her husband gifted me a beautiful, costly wristwatch and a gorgeous flower bouquet and requested a picture with his new 'bro-in-law'. As we had coffee in my office, I praised him via the interpreter and complimented his heroic struggle for his wife. I had seen many caring husbands; this one was the most loving. He looked at her, smiled, and turned to me. The interpreter translated his words again for me:

'Ducktoor, he says he will do it a hundred times again to see her healthy and happy. They will pray for you and your beloved every day'.

As they left, I remembered a moment in my childhood: lying down under the open sky upon our terrace, head upon my father's arm, both of us staring at the dark-blue enormity with diamonds sprinkled all across it. Baba had said, 'The only thing that defeats everything else in the world is immense love. Never fall short of it.'

I looked up at the sky again that night and smiled at my father.

He resonated in the sparkling stars and also in the dark-blue vastness of the sky.

CHAPTER 9

THE RENTAL GOONS WHOSE FATHER HAD AIDS

Admitted for treatment of memory loss, this big sixty-five-year-old man was found to be immunocompromised too; his HIV test had turned out positive. His memory loss was not typical, and he had developed fungal infection of the brain, common among the untreated immunocompromised patients.

He had four sons, all sturdy bodybuilders but very well-behaved with the hospital staff. They attended him religiously round the clock. They did not have a mother.

On the first day of his admission, I asked about his occupation. He was a renowned wrestler who had evolved into a hired bouncer and then recovery officer for private moneylenders. Upon losing his wife, he had continued to stay with his four sons, two of whom were married. They had accepted his regular guests, commercial sex workers, his only source of 'relaxation', as per the family.

Curious, I asked the elder son what he himself did for a living. Without any change in his expression or any body language that could suggest awkwardness, he replied, 'We four brothers have formed a company. People call us whenever they need to create problems . . . we can wash up anyone, start fights and even riots between political rivals. But we don't involve ourselves with criminal gangs or religious riots. We don't rob or steal. We just fight for salary.' I did not know whether to compliment that, so I stayed silent.

He opened up, happy that we were talking. 'We all graduated, sir. Baba has taken the best possible care of us all, he loves us very much. He encouraged us to eat well and go to the gym regularly. That's the reason we all are so strong. But we did not get any jobs with our degrees. People only offered us jobs as bouncers. Then we thought why work for others? So we opened this company. We are doing really good business.' He quoted some reputed names in social, business, and political spheres who were his clients and, in an attempt to impress me, also quoted some owners of academic institutions. 'Sometimes students, labour leaders, or rival parties trouble them, so they keep us on call . . . just like you are on call for hospital problems,' he added with a proud smile.

As the father was discharged, the two brothers took down notes about his diet, exercise, medicines, sleep, etc. Then the elder son asked if he could still avail of the HIV-positive commercial sex workers' services, both undergoing treatment.

We had involved an HIV specialist physician to counsel and advise them, so I batted that last question away to him. I had no academic, social, religious, moral, medical, or philosophical training to answer that question correctly then, at that point of time in my education.

While leaving, the son gave me his visiting card. 'Please call me if you ever need to. We have very high reach. We won't let anyone mess with you in Mumbai, take my word for it,' he said.

I did retain that card till I left India.

CHAPTER 10

THE BRAIN-ALIVE, HEART-DEAD

'We don't want her to suffer, Doc. We don't want any ventilator, etc., treatments,'

said the calm son, no traces of emotional tones in his speech. His seventy-two-year-old mother was admitted last night with stroke.

Quite a sophisticated family, this son owning a financial company of repute. His teenage daughter was sitting by her grandma in the ICU, patting her unconscious forehead.

'Can she hear us, Doctor?' the distraught granddaughter asked.

'Sometimes, only when she is a little more conscious.' It is difficult for me to be emotionally rude.

'Because I want to talk to her only once more . . . to say sorry. I was sulking after a fight with her when this happened. I should never have fought with her.' The sweet soul broke down.

Her father tried to calm her down, asked her to stop being too emotional about this and accept things like a mature grown-up. This is where I received the first shock. His pacifying his own daughter had a formality. It did not suggest 'I am proud of your emotional bond with my mother.' It, rather, suggested, 'Grow up, you stupid, these things happen.'

As I walked out of the ICU, his wife greeted me. 'How is Ma, Doc?' she asked.

I told her the truth: 'Fluctuating, but critical still.'

Then the expected question: 'How long, Doc? We don't want her to suffer too much.'

'Sorry, can't say at present.'

If I myself ever have an accident, I want to live. I want my doctor to try the best to make me survive, to give me one more chance to see and touch and hear my dear ones. I want to say sorry to those I may have offended and also to say proper goodbye to those who love me. I do not want my family to think about whether the doctors should try their best for me or not.

I have asked this very question to some people I have faith in the sanity of. The answer rarely was 'Don't save me if it took a lot of effort.' Some classified further: 'If I were to remain in a vegetative state permanently, only then, let go.'

Most of my old/very old patients explicitly state that they want to live as much as they can, with as much health that they can get. Nobody except the depressed/frustrated actually say that they want to die, a statement in itself contradictory to their being in the hospital.

I have had differences with some colleagues who 'let go' and encourage the willing family to make the same decision. It is useless, they argue, to spend so much and try for such a small possibility of meaningful survival. Patient must be able to choose dying with dignity, they advocate.

Many of my colleagues differ like myself and for a reason: if the patient has expressed a wish prior in complete senses that he/she wants no effort to be made for their survival, then a doctor must respect that. But I think *no* one else can make that decision on behalf of the patient after they have lost their senses without making such a decision. An unconscious patient is still alive until he/she is brain-dead, and it automatically becomes the duty of the doctor to make all efforts to try for the best outcome.

There are many sweet excuses people quote, including suffering, dignity, torture, tubes, pain, etc. to justify 'letting the patient die'. The real reasons often are expenses, time, hard work, stress, uncertainty associated with an elderly person being ill, and the perceived 'uselessness' of a debilitated/old/disabled person in the family, adding to the future bills. The elderly do not even have emotional value in many families now.

We are in a world where people have learnt the tact of carrying out entire discussions hypocritically, knowing that both are actually lying but still pretending to understand each other. Such 'manufactured' discussions decide the fates of hundreds of unfortunate old and unconscious patients who then become victims of 'lack-love' decisions made by the very people they gave birth to and grew up!

Expenses are a major issue in this decision-making. These can be reduced by offering care in smaller nursing homes/government hospitals. The nursing care decision of the vegetative patients almost always depends upon whether they will be useful to the society or not, whether they will earn and be productive again or not. For a world that calls itself civilised and developed, it is so primitive to let the elderly 'go' because they are now useless—that they have raised you and supported life when productive is not considered enough reason to nurse them well! The decision of whether the patient should be continued on life support or not should not be open for discussion if the patient has *not* written a will about it. If the patient is 'brain-alive', treatment must continue. For no team of neurologists/experts in the world will guarantee the outcome on the bad side: there are, many times, chances of regaining meaningful consciousness in every patient who is not brain-dead. And we, the living, who attempt every day taking whatever tiny chances we get to survive, to grope more and more of life we can, should be the last people to say 'Let go' when it comes to someone else's life. It would morally amount to a murder.

'We hear some doctors keep dead bodies on ventilator in the ICU just to extract more money,' said one business-minded friend to me once, after watching some cheap populist movie. We doctors are well-trained against violence, so I answered him verbally only: 'With all hospitals almost running full, critical patients in waiting areas, why would any hospital keep on ventilating the dead?'

There are monitors, files, paperwork, and many doctors, nurses, and other staff in each critical care unit. How can people imagine that the dead will be kept on machines in such units? Or is it just another social trick to mask the mirror of reality? A small question: if the hospitals start declaring all who chose to 'shut down' life support systems upon their own relatives/parents, took such critical patients home, or admitted them late beyond life-saving period, will our society be happy about it? Then why make such gruesome allegations against a whole profession who even bring some dead back with immense effort without even knowing them? Why do you think thousands of Code Blue teams run without caring for their own life when someone is dying, anywhere in the world?

There are also many relatives who don't sleep, don't even eat till their patient regains consciousness. There are many who silently suffer with the patient. Many sell their belongings to pay hospital bills and still tell the doctor, 'Try your best, Doctor *saab*, don't worry about anything. I will pay every bill.'

These two—the doctors and relatives who try to save the critical, especially old, patients desperately—are both being classified under 'impractical, stupid' people gradually.

Because our society has matured to money.

As I met the patient next day, still in the twilight zone between life and death, there was no one with her except the granddaughter with swollen eyes. She exclaimed, smiling through her tears, 'Doc, she opened her eyes and looked at me for a few seconds. She didn't say anything, but I knew she recognised me and she was happy to see me. I know her eyes. She was awake in that moment.' And she broke into sobs.

Mercy in the skies often comes alive only with love.

The patient regained her senses in a week.

As she asked for discharge, holding her granddaughter's hand, she looked at her son standing by and proudly told me, 'Doc, this is my son. He owns the XYZ Company. He takes very good care of me.'

Avoiding eye contact with anyone, he hugged his mother and said, 'I love you, Ma.'

His teenage daughter kept staring at the floor. I looked at her face.

I don't wish to see that extremely scary expression again.

CHAPTER 11

SEX? SHUT UP!

They married in love, both highly placed software professionals. Their families didn't agree, so they chose to stay away from their parents in a different city and had a sweet daughter soon after. Ties with parents resumed to formalities.

She developed a neurological problem and became almost crippled at an early age of twenty-eight. She also lost bladder and bowel control and became diaper dependent. He now took care of her and the daughter, struggling to cope up with his job responsibilities. To save, he cooked at home often. Parents on both sides refused to assist in any way. He had thus been tied up 24/7 since the last five years, and I witnessed the downfall of a normal, happy man alongside the medical tragedy that unfolded upon his wife. 'She would also have cared the same for me if this had happened to me,' he said.

They could not have proper sex due to her medical condition. He did not want to deceive her.

Last time, he broke down, talking alone to me. 'Sir, people offer weird suggestions. I want to have normal sex. I have been starving for the last six years. I don't know what to do. Is it abnormal if I want to feel physical love? I can't divorce her as even her parents have given her up, and I cannot even talk about this to her—it will hurt her. Saints, law, society all advise so many things otherwise but don't guide in my situation. It is very easy to advise celibacy to others. It was never my wish, so I cannot accept that lifestyle.

'I was so full of life once. I am all suffocated now. There is no solution. Even talking about sex is a taboo in our country.'

I was used to the 'relationship' concept in the developed world, where breaking up of a couple was better accepted after the diagnosis of an incurable disease than in India, and sex was not looked down upon when others had it by choice. But any suggestions offered in this case would have been classified as 'immoral' or 'illegal' in India. A recent high-court judgment even equated one-time sex with marriage and the compulsion thereof.

'One must find personal solace' was all that I could tell him, besides comforting him with kind words.

This affects many women and men, due to physical or mental illness, superstition (guilt about having sexual feelings), or accidents. Some realise impotence or incurable sexual abnormalities of their partner only after the marriage and are doomed to an almost sexless life. There are many clinics/specialists who can help some, but this mostly goes on as an inevitable, relentless suffering. Their cross is the perpetual answer, 'Shut up and kill your desire,' from almost everyone. Many Indian parents still look down upon their grown-up children who discuss sex. Most merchants of morals disappear from this scene. Law has no answers; it is only judgmental about this. Intellectuals use wise, philosophical wordplay but don't dare to answer straight.

The answers are not difficult; the courage to word them is lacking.

CHAPTER 12

THE JOURNEY IN PAIN

'Will I ever win? I feel suicidal,' said the twenty-five-year-old orphan with multiple sclerosis. In a world drooling over the stories of 'Ten Richest' or 'Twenty Most Beautiful' women, there's hardly any scope for noticing an orphan girl who fights alone against an incurable disease.

Veena, a dignified young Indian lady, divides her life fighting three wars: living as a single female at a bed-share facility for women, working her job as a receptionist at a nearby clinic that earns her a minor income, and the incurable neurological disease, multiple sclerosis that causes disability at an early age.

'My mother left me at an orphanage when I was two years old. She saw me last when I was three. After that, I don't know anything about her or my father. The orphanage taught me how to survive with wild human beings around. They also helped for my education. I was diagnosed with MS when I was twenty. They shifted me to Pune for better climate. Now I am pursuing a BA,' Veena told me.

'The owner of the orphanage in Pune didn't know multiple sclerosis and always said I was faking my limp and fatigue. She made me do a lot of physical work. I couldn't. So I left that orphanage.'

She then stayed at various places: a blind school where a volunteer was required, homes of other MS patients who came to know her through the MS society, sometimes on the streets, and now got a bed share at a dingy, cramped female hostel.

'Whenever I get sick and cannot walk due to MS attack, a local hospital helps me with steroid doses, the MS society gives some medicines free. Sometimes other MS patients pay for my treatment'.

Now she has developed mood swings and depression, common in MS patients, especially those her age. Naturally, her behaviour is intolerable or unacceptable to those who invite her to stay with them. Where we cannot tolerate the raised voice and mental fluctuations of our own parents and children, who is trained to shoulder those of an orphan? Who will pause their own life to feel the dying mental pulse of someone who knows that there will be no one to look after her if at all she is crippled and that there is no cure for her illness yet?

No language in this world can truly describe loneliness.

'Some societies help, but they have their rules. The MS society helped me many times. But then, how long can I do this?' She is now tired. She knows her limp will not improve. She knows free treatments are not the only answer. 'I feel suicidal often now. I know things will never be my way. Life will always be at the mercy of someone's help.'

I told her it is common to feel so in MS and that good treatments and counselling can help most patients.

Her reply left me shut: 'Sir, I don't need that. I plan to fight this with my own mind, for I want to survive without any mental dependence. Someone should have counselled my mother when she dumped me. I wanted to marry and have children. Who will marry me? I know I am beautiful and some men are after me, but none for marrying.' These are probably the most difficult words for a proud woman to say to anyone, and her eyes clouded red.

As Veena broke down in a tearless silence, I fought with a hundred false reassuring words I could say. I didn't want to insult her suffering by saying them. A doctor must learn to cry within, still with a smile upon his face.

I remembered the story about Lord Jesus Christ, describing his *via dolorosa* (journey of pain) when he had to carry his own cross while being tortured all the way to the site of his own crucifixion.

There are so many patients who know they are going downhill, that they will never return to good life again. No songs of motivation, no thunderous clapping of groups, no shouting of any slogans, no celebrations of their plight will ever cure them. Our world is addicted to superficial, temporary relief in an attempt of self-glorification at the cost of someone else's suffering. Genuine help is rare; charity show-offs make it big.

Real answers are far away.

So much so that a country that plans multi-crore space missions in search of new life cannot take care of the live suffering of a young woman existing *now*, here, amongst us! A country proud of one-hundred-crore-worth movies and billion-dollar IPLs cannot support its own daughter in suffering.

There is no hope for dignity without money.

An orphan is as much a social and national responsibility as environment or defence.

And these words are just screams in a black hole!

God, solve this please.

CHAPTER 13

A MURDERER WHO ALMOST KILLED US

The whole city awaited a murder, just like in the book *Chronicle of a Death Foretold* by Mr Gabriel Garcia Marquez.

It was 1992. I was posted in the casualty along with Dr Anwar and Dr Junaid, my batchmates. The postings were phenomenal in that we got hands-on experience on a variety of medical emergencies.

There had been a murder in the city few days ago, a result of a professional rivalry between two big families. One was shot point-blank in cold blood on a busy street. The brother of the dead had sworn that he would kill the killer soon. It was just a question of time. The anxiety was subtly in the air for a few days.

We had our customary 2 a.m. tea at the tea shop on the street opposite the hospital and were just re-entering the casualty when there were panicked screams outside and a whole lot of people barged in, asking for the doctor on duty. Dr Anwar said that the medical officer was in his room and asked about the patient.

The patient was the victim's brother, the one who had sworn to kill the murderer. He had developed severe vomiting and diarrhoea and had become unconscious. He also heavily smelt of alcohol. The medical officer on duty, a skin specialist, came over. He examined the patient and ordered medical tests, including blood alcohol levels and the analysis of stomach aspirate. Writing the treatment plan, he told us to carry it out and left to retire.

I looked for a good vein to start the IV fluids. Dr Junaid recorded the pulse and BP, both a little out of range but acceptable. I got the vein. We gave him the advised medicines. The patient was stable.

Dr Anwar started to write the police a note: We must inform all medicolegal cases in hospital campus immediately to the police.

Dr Junaid whispered to me, 'Some relatives smelt of probably marijuana.'

It was a cubicle, the dressing room beside inpatient casualty, made of government-grade cheap plywood, with a table and chair, patient bed, IV stand, and an elementary dressing cart. It had only one door, blocked by at least twenty relatives, all shouting angrily about why the patient was still unconscious. 'If something happens to him, you will not survive,' some of them kept on repeating. They were headed by an extremely aggressive and big lady, who said she was the patient's sister. We told her he was stable and expected to improve.

'Why isn't he conscious yet?' she asked angrily.

We started getting anxious.

The security guards were meekly standing behind the crowd. They were both government servants, and this crowd was above them and even the government, knowing who was who.

The telephone rang. It was the hospital's ambulance driver, our night-tea partner, calling from a ward. He said in a hurried and anxious voice, 'Sir, they are not good people. Leave that room. I will keep the ambulance ready outside if you want to come out. Don't argue with them,' he said.

'We cannot,' I said. The relatives were right there.

'We need some IV fluids,' I told him.

'Yes, sir.' He got it.

Dr Anwar handed over the police information sheet to a ward boy waiting out, through the crowd.

The patient's sister snatched it from his hand. 'What is this?' she asked.

'The senior doctor asked us to file an MLC [medicolegal case] as there is suspicion of alcohol intoxication and food poisoning,' explained Dr Anwar, carefully choosing his words but still with hesitation. It is never easy to talk peacefully to someone angry and aggressive.

Then there was a loud noise, a wet and heavy and muffled thud. She had slapped Dr Anwar. 'My brother is dying, and you want to file a police case?' She caught hold of his shirt collar and bent and lifted him with her hand between his legs, kicking him all the while. Dr Junaid and I ran to her, saying many things that meant sorry, it was just a procedure, we had been ordered by our senior, her brother was not dying but stable, etc. You know how coherent one can be in such a situation.

We were pushed back violently by the crowd then. 'You don't move from here till our brother is conscious,' we were told, with added expletives.

The aggressive lady lifted up Dr Anwar and banged him on the plywood. It gave way, shattering also the glass with it. Dr Anwar started shouting for help as she continued to fist and kick him. One relative lifted up the chair and started breaking the telephone and the glass on the cubicle walls and then aimed at us. We begged him not to throw the chair. He did anyway, and we turned away to dodge that chair. The metal bruised Dr Junaid's ear and my arm; we both started bleeding. More fists and kicks fell upon us.

The patient moved, pulled out his IV line. Blood started soaking the white bed sheet. Just as I moved to get a syringe to temporarily block it (it was an open needle), someone slapped my back. 'Can't you see he is bleeding? Stop it.' Dr Junaid reconnected the IV line with bare hands, trembling.

At this point, the civil surgeon entered, an old man with many political and social connections. He was accompanied by two to three police constables and the senior doctor on duty who had called them. The family knew the CS. He pacified them, told them he will look after the patient personally, and asked them all to go to his room.

The in-charge sister, a locum mother to us all, took us to the doctor's room and dressed our wounds. The ambulance driver got us some coffee.

The CS never asked us if we were hurt. He kept on telling the stories of how he calmed down the crowd for ages later. He never felt responsible for what happened nor reprimanded his 'friends' for their violent behaviour with his junior doctors.

The patient improved and was discharged in three days. The whole family came to take him away again. They left without any thanks or apologies. Someone who had openly declared that he was going to kill another walked out of the hospital, face up, with friends and family. A violent family that had attacked the very doctors treating him.

About a week later, the patient fulfilled what he had promised his family: he killed his brother's murderer in open daylight, witnessed by dozens on a busy city square.

Dr Anwar and Dr Junaid have long left India and are happily settled in safer countries.

Twenty years down the line, I continue to read the same story almost every day in India.

CHAPTER 14

THE MADMAN

Time and again, relatives dump the invalid, disabled, psychotic, or infectious patients in a government hospital, provide false addresses or names, and disappear. By default, the ward staff (mainly nurses, ward boys, and resident doctors) look after such patients. There are some 'local tricks' we have to help these patients stay till some option is arranged (finding out a relative by involving police or social worker or shifting them to a ward where there are vacancies, etc.). Almost every doctor who studied in India has spent for such patients from his or her pocket; that too umpteen times—for their medicines (which are never available in required quantity at any government hospital), tea, etc., often sharing home food with them.

An absolutely disoriented, violent, and sturdy young man in his twenties was admitted one Friday in the psychiatry ward via casualty. No police or relatives accompanied him, and no history was available. When I first met him, he was restrained (hands and legs tied down to the bed) and shouting in spite of the injectable sedatives and antipsychotics he was given. He refused to talk; we tried different languages. I called my lecturer, who told me there was nothing more to be done, as higher doses could cause respiratory paralysis, and as there was no ICU or ventilator, I would have to intubate him and sit by his side with an ambu bag to ventilate him all night.

I had had my first son just a few weeks ago. Being my son, he was genetically nocturnal, and so it was my duty to look after him all night till he slept in the early morning. He preferred that I carried him in my arms and walked through the hostel's dark corridors and would start an agitation if I sat down. So I could not stay out of the hostel at night.

As the patient refused to eat and didn't touch his food, I asked the nurse to start IV fluids for that day (he wouldn't allow a feeding tube).

The next morning, around 9 a.m., my lecturer took rounds and plainly instructed us that as soon as he was calmer, we had to discharge him. 'If something happens in the ward or he runs away and harms anyone, we'll have to spend a lot of time in silly, stupid, mindless paperwork and enquiries,' he said. He had a point there.

'But sir, he has no relatives. Where will he go?' I asked.

'You take him home. He will feel at home with you,' my lecturer commented with a big devil smile, as my colleagues laughed aloud. They had found their gossip topic for next few days. Dissent is killed in medicine with cruel sarcasm all over the world; we must all grow up with this.

At 5 p.m. that day, I got a call from the nurse; the patient had run away when she had untied him to go to the washroom with a servant. I informed the lecturer, who said unprintable things in his local rural mother tongue directed towards the patient and, in general, his own job. 'Inform police,' he said at the end of his brief sparkling monologue about life.

I took my scooter and went to the ward. Informed police. The nurse was terrified; she told me he had run away towards the hostels.

Although dirty and not maintained, most govt. hospital campuses are big. GHATI in Aurangabad, where I was training for MD, was super big, over ten acres, with multiple ward buildings a huge college building and staff quarters. I decided to give it a try and went on searching every road.

I found him sitting upon a large stone in the big ground behind staff quarters, an isolated area covered with grass. Parking my scooter, I went to him. He saw me but didn't react. I sat near him and asked him questions softly. He kept looking away. Then I just sat there. The sun started downing.

'I am hungry', he said in Hindi, all of a sudden.

'OK. Five minutes. Stay here, I will get you something,' I said and ran. Proud of my speed on the scooter, I broke my own records that day and reached our college canteen.

Our eternal food god, Mr Sundar Anna, who managed the college canteen, knew hundreds of budding doctors by name. He had to keep accounts and use funny sounding threats in his Malayalam-accented Hindi to stop giving them food if they did not pay the bills. (This he never did.) He took my order with a masked face (I was overdue eighty rupees by then, and he would next smile at me only when and if I paid it). He reminded me of the total in stern tones as I took the parcel. 'Sorry Sundar Anna, I'm a little short of funds this week,' I told him, making an innocent face. He looked away too.

Our patient was still there. He took the pastry and ate it. He threw away the other dish without tasting it.

'Come to the ward. It will be cold out here—you cannot sleep here. Also, there are many insects and mosquitoes here,' I requested him.

'They tied me to the bed,' he complained. I reassured him that now they wouldn't.

He got up and walked with me to the ward. The nurse was ever happy. I continued my ward work with other patients.

When the ward boy brought him dinner, he kept staring at that food.

It is beyond us to understand why we do some things instinctively. Just having had a son myself, I was all of a father at age twenty-three, and that spirit is divine. I picked up a morsel from his plate and held it to his mouth. He ate it. As the tearful nurse watched us with water in her hands, he ate a complete dinner that night like a child, as I fed him morsel after morsel. Somehow we were not afraid of him now.

This was so rewardingly peaceful to my soul. I thought it was gifted by the universe with some purpose. I understood it much later: that no one is insane at all times. If you reach the correct point and time, everyone is amenable to love. You must possess it at all times for it to work.

It was the most beautiful thing I learnt as a doctor.

He improved. His name was Ramsukh; he was from a northern state called Uttar Pradesh. He had run away from his home, as his parents had not allowed him to marry his love. The girl was married to someone else due to the pressures of their community. They had threatened to kill him if he revolted against the community. He remembered getting in a state transport bus from Mumbai to our city but nothing after that.

He was discharged in a few weeks. By then, he had regained a narrow-minded sanity that this society could grasp.

CHAPTER 15

THE SHOCKING ILLNESS

The young and disturbed couple sat in front of me, avoiding eye contact. They were embarrassed and angry at each other and hesitant as to who should start. The man was almost a giant, six foot three, and very well built (he was a professional gym instructor). The wife was athletic but of average height.

Finally, the lady gathered courage.

'It was our wedding night, Doctor, a year ago. We slept at about three in the morning. At about 4 a.m., he suddenly got out of the bed and screamed so loud that I was frightened. I thought he had hurt himself somewhere. I asked him what happened, but he didn't recognise me and looked at me as if I was a stranger. I was dead scared. I ran out and called his parents. He didn't even recognise his father. When the fifty-five–year-old father held his hand and told him to sit down, he lifted up his father and banged him head down upon the floor. He then kept shouting and randomly moving through the house. His mom and myself, we stayed away, watching him, but he never looked at us or said anything. After some time, he came to the bed and slept. I was never scared so much earlier. His father had a bad head injury and had to be operated upon. We told at the hospital that he had fallen down to avoid a police case. My husband (the patient) does not remember anything. I can't believe it.'

'We consulted a psychiatrist, and he got my husband investigated. He said it was due to stress and gave an antidepressant, which my husband stopped in few months. After a few months, the same thing repeated. I was the victim—fortunately, I only fractured a hand. It happened almost at the same time early morning. Then we went to a neurologist. We were told that he had a rare type of epilepsy called complex partial seizures (CPS). But even with treatment for this, he has had three such attacks.'

'I don't know what to do. I cannot sleep out of fear. He says he doesn't know what he is doing in that phase. It is not his mistake. I want to believe him but cannot. He does not drink or smoke and takes good care of us all. I know he loves me very much, but I am always scared of him.'

The embarrassed and extremely awkward patient tried to explain to me how he did not really understand or remember what happened in those moments when he was violent. The poor man came to tears, guilty about what he had done to his family. Their marriage was on a shaky edge.

Upon questioning, he revealed that he had had fits during fever (febrile seizures) in his childhood. This is known to lead to some minor or major damage in a part of the brain called the hippocampus. This damage causes sudden bursts of electrical surges in the brain, leading to episodes of abnormal behaviour or convulsions, which are called CPS. Patient does not remember most of these. These may range from very minor, unnoticeable behaviours like repetitive blinking, lip smacking, rocking, etc., to such severe forms as narrated above. Physical examination is mostly normal in such cases, and some tests may confirm the diagnosis.

Some external factors may lead to generation of such abnormal discharges. The most common ones are fever, fasting, lack of sleep, and some medicines. In this case, lack of sleep was an association. With dose adjustment and proper sleep, he has kept well for last few years now.

CPS is a very intriguing type of epilepsy, which causes sudden abnormal/repetitive/patterned behaviour lasting a few seconds to minutes. Patients may behave extremely irrationally. There are cases who suddenly become fearful and catch hold of person standing next to them, speak gibberish, or perform meaningless actions/gestures. Some behave confused or start shouting aloud. Some stumble, giving an impression of being drunk. In a predominantly illiterate, superstitious country like India, they are unfortunately often roughed up for such behaviour. Many times we have had such patients in casualty: badly beaten up by the macho men searching for a chance to exhibit their heroic muscles, brought by police or public, who tell that the patient was 'misbehaving'. Careful analysis reveals the truth, and patients often reveal that they had been beaten up or punished even prior for their epilepsy.

Some patients may have many types of fits—the ones described above and also convulsions. Epilepsy patients sometimes suffer depression or psychosis. On multiple medicines, some may develop complex behavioural problems. A good neurologist and psychiatrist can together solve these issues successfully in most cases. Some cases benefit with surgery.

While such patients should not drive or swim, many are unaware of this illness. If the diagnosis is confirmed, any new medicines for any other illness must be cross-checked for its likelihood of causing fits. Most patients, once diagnosed and explained well, can lead a completely normal and productive life.

CHAPTER 16

THE BEAUTY AND THE HORROR: PART I

'You are posted in the mobile hospital next month onwards for three months. It is near Kannad Village this summer.' I was told by the clerk who conveyed postings to the intern doctors. Adventurous inside, I was excited and told my friends about my new posting.

'You are screwed' was their universal opinion.

These postings were usually in the remote interiors, far away from any city. No entertainment, no guarantee of good food, and usually mosquito-studded nights. Most dangerously, everyone posted usually left for home on Thursday, leaving the juniormost intern alone for next three days to attend the rural, uneducated populace with basic minimum facility: a midwife (dai) who doubled as a nurse and a few servants to assist. The leftover medicines and syringes, IV fluids, etc. donated by the world for the famous Kumbh-Mela, a gathering of millions of devotees in India, and other occasions, were used in this clinic. Wards, minor OT, labour room, pantry . . . all in tents carried around by a caravan of four huge trucks.

After three hours of travel, a bus dropped me near the village, and I walked in the only direction that the road went ahead of there. I saw the trucks parked in a school ground and a banner upon one of them: Mobile Hospital. A school that had closed down for lack of funds was emptied for us: seven rooms, mostly without doors or windowpanes but with metal cots upon which we could sleep and a common roofless bathroom. A nearby sugar factory had agreed to offer meals and breakfast to all posted doctors free; we just had to walk to their campus canteen a mile away. Thank God!

But I was alone. Even my in-charge medical officer was not there yet. The first two days, I worked with the servants to set up, helping wherever I could. As always, I had carried my Ayn Rand and Richard Bach with me, and also my notebook to write poems (there is no treatment for this disorder of writing poetry). It was a welcome break, wandering in raw, wet green farmlands far away and then returning at dinner time, jumping lifts in bullock carts! Zen atmosphere!

On the third morning, just as I finished breakfast and returned to the hospital, the servant told me one of my superiors had arrived. I ran to the office.

'Hi!' said the most beautiful face I had ever seen.

Fair, curly brown hair tossed back neatly; big hazel sunshine eyes; radiant, beautiful face,; the grace of a princess; and the sweetest way of carrying herself— she had a smile that instantly disoriented me. She was simply mesmerizing. I already had a crush, damn it!

'How are you, Mr Poet?' she asked, and I blushed. Thinking that no one would touch it, I had left my notebook in the office where I had sat writing last evening.

'I'm Dr Rajas,' I told her. No intern (or higher qualified doctor) usually misses a chance of adding the prefix *Dr* to their name whenever they can, especially in this situation. Then it becomes a habit!

'Yes, I know you. I saw you on stage in that annual day drama where you played the spoiled medical student. Didn't you feel awkward and scared to hold that magazine on the stage? All our teachers were there.' she asked, with pretend anger. I receded into dark shame zone; it must have shown upon my mug.

'Hey, I am joking. I liked that play and your act too. I am Sharayu,' she said. 'I am third-year PG and exam-going. I'll depend upon you for my study. I've got my books with me. I will just attend the OB-GY patients and deliveries if any. Okay?'

'Yes, ma'am.' She was three years older!

So what?

Patients had started walking in, so we got busy.

At lunch, she told me two more colleagues were coming for the posting after three days: a surgeon and a physician.

As we walked back after lunch, she kept talking about what she had studied yesterday. Her speech to me was like a flute: sweet, meaningless, but a soothing melody.

She studied the whole day. I pined for the evening, when I could talk again with her.

At around five, I finished OPD and made tea for her in our pantry tent. She was probably used to this kind of treatment and people being fascinated with her.

She drank *my* tea with pleased dimples that bejewelled her face.

'Let's go for a walk,' she said, and we wandered into the farms, walking over the weirs between farms, often holding hands to support each other. The sparkling evening skies were the colour of pink champagne, and the grounds were all wet and soft, deep emerald. That evening is frozen in my mind. We made instant friends and clicked like magnets. We talked about so many things and returned to the factory to have dinner.

We played cards till late night, and she went to sleep in the next room with the nurse.

I sat outside in the big, breezy ground and lighted my favourite. This was one of the best days in life yet, and it called for a celebration. How sarcastic is fate that the happiest moments in life cannot be shared with anyone; they demand loneliness as their price! I went in my room long after midnight.

The candlelight in the room started playing with the shadows it had created, moving them to the tunes of the breezes.

'Hey,' she said from the open door. 'Awake yet? Can't sleep?'

'Don't want to. Very happy. Come in.'

'I want to see you write a poem,' she said.

'Have a seat,' I said, offering her a broken but workable chair from my palace. 'Why? Don't you believe I can write?'

'I know you can, and I read a little from your notebook. I'm sorry, but I liked them.' She winked. 'I just want to see you write them.'

'Okay.' I sat down beside her.

The breezes became jealous and started blowing wild whistles.

'What do you want me to write a poem about?' I asked her.

'Me.' And she smiled, again disorienting me. 'Or anything,' she corrected.

I scribbled some drunken lines about how I felt when I looked at her.

She read it with intense eyes. She was not smiling when she looked up.

She ruffled my hair. 'I like you too—you are a sweetheart. Remember, I must also concentrate on my studies. We have a few days to be together. I want to talk to you so much!'

'Come out,' I said.

There, among the bright moon, the starry sky, and the breezy night, we sat upon the school stairs holding hands, talking about nothing, till the skies started to wake up in their baby-orange overalls.

Wishing each other a good night at early morning, we went in to sleep.

Who could imagine what horror was on the way!

CHAPTER 17

THE BEAUTY AND THE HORROR: PART II

The morning began beautifully again. I woke her up around eight, and she wished me a good morning in a honeyed sleepy smile. Dressed up, we had tea together. She taught me some topic she had studied yesterday. Flute again.

By noon, there were three admissions. One boy who fell from a tree and had a head injury and vomited but was stable. Second was an elderly patient with an asthma attack, and the third was a twenty-eight-year-old lady with high-grade fever. While the other two had stabilised well, the lady had started getting delirious already. Fever, chills, rigors, typical malarial pattern in a region where malaria was a dreaded killer. She was pregnant—three months. The man accompanying her, a distant cousin, told us that her husband stayed in another village.

I called upon Dr Sharayu. After examining the patient, she called the in-charge medical officer who was still on leave and talked to him on the phone. He advised to shift the patient to the nearest rural hospital a few miles away, but her cousin said they had no means to travel and asked us to do what best we could. As per the senior MO's advice, she prescribed injectable paracetamol and oral chloroquine along with antacids to this patient. These were the only options available with us. The lady stabilised by the next day, her delirium was reversed and fever subsided. She ate well, and her vitals were normal.

The second day with Dr Sharayu was as beautiful as the first. We walked around the campus, talking about so many things but mostly books and music. Just as we returned after the dinner, the nurse told us that the admitted lady had pain in the lower abdomen. Dr Sharayu examined her in privacy and told me there was a possibility she might abort and she needed to be shifted to a higher centre with ultrasonography, OT, and better care in case there was severe bleeding. We also did not have the necessary medicines there to prevent abortion.

A farmer who was returning from the sugar factory in his small truck agreed to help us take her to the nearest rural hospital about five miles away. Both me and Dr Sharayu went with the patient and her cousin to the RH. We reached there by 9 p.m. and found that the medical officer there, Dr Hante, was an ill-behaved, irritable, short, and bulky man who was already drunk and talked with a lot of tobacco in his mouth. We introduced ourselves. As Dr Sharayu narrated him the case, he kept on scanning her. He did not ask her to sit down. In a few minutes, Dr Sharayu realised that he was all lust and then told me in a whisper to stay put beside her at all times. The farmer with the truck waited for us to return.

Dr Hante got the patient admitted. Then turning to me, he said I could go back to the mobile hospital and that Dr Sharayu will have to stay there.

'Why?' she asked.

He asked me to go with the patient to the ward for admission.

'No, sir, I will stay here. I don't know what I can do with the patient now,' I said.

He turned at me, all vicious. 'Too smart, are you?' he asked. 'You must listen to your seniors,' he said.

'She is my senior, sir, I am posted with her,' I said firmly.

He then asked the witnessing relatives and other staff to leave.

He turned to Dr Sharayu. 'Tell your intern to leave,' he told her.

Innocent and frightened but hiding it, she asked, 'Why, sir? What am I needed here for now? You are such a senior and experienced OB-GY specialist. I know you can take care of her better than me. Plus I am feeling feverish. I would like to go back and sleep.'

'Don't worry, I will arrange a room here if you are unwell,' he said.

'Sorry, sir. I think I will leave now with Dr Rajas,' Dr Sharayu said.

Then he unveiled the snakes hidden in his mind. 'Look here, Sharayu. The patient may abort. I can tell them that you gave her a wrong medicine. These people are illiterate and very dangerous. You will never know what happened to you. Just listen to what I tell you.'

I looked around for things that could make a weapon. Just in case.

'But what wrong medicine? Chloroquine and paracetamol are both safe in pregnancy. I talked to the person in charge before starting these,' Dr Sharayu flared up.

'Chloroquine can cause abortion sometimes,' he said.

'So can high-grade fever. There was no option but to give chloroquine. She would have died otherwise,' she retorted.

'They will listen to me, not you. Now don't argue—it will not be safe for you,' he concluded.

'I will stay with her if she must stay here,' I said, and before the angry Dr Hante could say anything, Dr Sharayu said in a calm, firm, raised voice, 'No, Rajas. We are leaving. I know we have done nothing wrong.' She started walking out.

He stood in the door.

'You are exam-going. I know your internal examiners well. I am going to tell them that you misbehaved,' he said. Then he added, 'You misunderstand, Dr Sharayu. I will need your help in case this patient requires some intervention.'

Dr Sharayu, too hurt and angry to answer, held my hands while standing behind me and walked out of the door, dodging him.

The truck-driver farmer was waiting. We were surprised to find him angry too. 'I heard what he said, madam. This doctor is a known alcoholic and womaniser, madam—ignore him. Do you have people at your mobile hospital, or do you want me to stay there tonight? I will sleep in my truck outside,' he offered.

'No, we have some staff there.' We thanked him.

The next morning, just after breakfast, the patient's cousin came in with three other men, two clad in white kurta, a trademark of sociopolitical nuisance now. The third one appeared to be a shady bearded farmer.

I sat beside Dr Sharayu.

'Our patient aborted yesterday,' the shady one said. 'You gave her wrong medicines.'

Dr Sharayu smiled bravely and told them, 'Look, *bhaiya* [brother], the medicines were not wrong. If we didn't use them, she might have died. In fact, she was better the next day only because of treatment.'

'We don't understand that,' said one white kurta. 'We plan to file a police case.'

We both didn't know what to answer. We called the nurse, an elderly lady. She told the relatives that this was the standard treatment and that the other medical officer was trying to take advantage of the situation.

They laughed. 'We've known him for many years now. He is our friend. He will never do anything wrong.'

Dr Sharayu became tearful. 'Do what you want,' she said and got up.

The second in a white kurta spoke. 'Don't cry, Doctor. We will find some way. These are illiterate, poor idiots. We will manage them.' He touched her shoulder.

The nurse removed his hand from Dr Sharayu's shoulder. 'It's okay, you go and do what you want. We will call our medical officer in charge.' she told the white kurta who was already almost drooling.

They left but stayed parked in their tractor right in front of the school.

The staff grouped around us. 'Leave as fast as possible. These people mean trouble,' they told us.

How?

I walked with her to the factory. The tractor followed us slowly. We requested the cook to please allow us a phone call. He did. We called our medical officer in charge and narrated what had happened.

'Don't worry, I will be there tomorrow morning,' he said. 'Stay together.'

As we washed hands in the isolated area behind the dining room, Dr Sharayu broke down. 'I am very scared,' she said.

I reassured her, 'Don't worry, I will not let them harm you.' I meant it.

We walked back, stalked again.

As we entered the school ground at around 2 p.m., a glistening white Maruti Gypsy car entered the campus. 'Hi, Sharayu!' cried someone from the driver's seat.

They were the remaining two PGs, the medicine and surgery residents. One of them, if I remember correctly, was one Dr M. Menon. They had come to stay for the posting.

We came to life again and told them what all had happened in the last two days. They were already among Dr Sharayu's fans and came out with the expected surgical response: 'Let's go beat them up'.

'No, we are among strangers. Can it,' said Dr Sharayu.

'Come, let's go get some tea,' the medical resident said. We paused in front of the tractor, making loud, manly conversations about what could happen if anyone tried funny stuff with us.

By the time we returned, they had left. We finished the waiting OPD and spent a disturbed night awake. The next morning, our in-charge came. He had already met the infamous Dr Hante on his way to us and exchanged threats, saying that if at all anyone was wrong, it was his responsibility, and if Dr Hante dared to create a nuisance, his fitness and habits too would be complained against. That resolved the issue.

The whole team went away after three days. Our in-charge met the local Sarpanch (sociopolitical head), and we were assured security via nearby resident villagers.

I spent one of the most beautiful months of my life then, in that heaven. The kind of heaven that is heaven because there is this one person you want in it.

CHAPTER 18

THE MOST HORRIBLE DAYS AS A DOCTOR: PART I

'Ready?'

As I held the knife, Dr PTJ said, 'Hold the knife like a pen, keep the tip on the skin, and with a controlled but firm pressure downwards, confidently swipe its edge down as you feel the skin resistance. Don't go deep at all. I am here. Start.'

Sweating a little, I prayed and looked down at the exposed abdomen in front of me. It moved passively, slowly, breathing, albeit tense. Everyone waited impatiently. Dr PTJ was known to be short-tempered even by surgeons' standards.

As I cut open the first live human body, tiny spurts of blood oozed out; he wiped them.

This is the second take-off in surgery; the first one starts when the patient is anaesthetised. I kept on assisting Dr PTJ as he opened different layers of the abdomen below the skin, stopping the bleeding at each level. He opened the innermost layer called the peritoneum, and the swollen intestines, purplish-black by now, popped out. He showed me how to clamp the swollen part at both ends and cut it open, clear the gangrenous dead parts, and suture the open ends in layers. That surgery of a complicated intestinal obstruction took above three hours. During pauses, he showed me the 'danger areas' where one could cause fatal bleeding. He then taught me the stitching back of abdomen in layers.

One life was saved in over a thousand steps, I was euphoric like a child. I had done nothing major, but the seniors still praised, maybe just to encourage. Looking at my face, Dr PTJ joked, 'You cannot smile until the patient is discharged.' I thanked him and went out.

It was 11 a.m. Ecstatic, I went out with my friend Manoj for a smoke and a tea. A casualty servant came rushing there. 'Sir, come to casualty—fast.' I ran, leaving Manoj alone.

There was chaos. The police had brought four cases of stabbing in a religious riot. There was blood all over the floor. Dr PTJ was shouting, 'Call the other three surgeons and anaesthetists. One stay here. Rajas, you check vitals, start IV, and put in a feeding tube, send blood for grouping and lab, then wait till the anaesthetist gives fitness. When your reliever comes here, you join me in OT.' He was tense.

One of the new patients had already arrested (no heart sounds), so the other intern was performing CPR upon him. There was only one working curtain stand in the casualty, now occupied by a dead body. So everyone else, including other patients and relatives, could see the CPR, where the chest massage caused oozing of blood from the abdominal wounds.

The other three were all in shock—very low BP, bleeding from chest or abdomen. Just as we finished starting IV lines and covering the bleeding wounds, ordering blood sampling and ECGs, another ambulance came over with six more. In next five hours, over thirty patients filled up the ten bedded casualty, stabbed or shot. Some came in pairs, having stabbed each other. Some were brought in dead. The casualty floor was all blood. Every medical officer, intern, nurse, and ward boy was in the hospital, working on their best steam. The blood bank techs were about to faint.

I went to the OT. Four of the surgeons were operating already with combined staff. They were from different religions, including the communities fighting outside. Dr PTJ and Dr AM, with whom I was posted, both sobbed as they operated. They knew the outcomes when they opened the abdomen.

The rioters had used swords, knives, blunt rods, almost anything for stabbing. But where there was a sword or knife used, some had not only stabbed but they had also rotated the weapon's blade inside the victim, thus cutting many vital organs like the liver, spleen, lungs, and blood vessels. Intestines were cut open in many places. In most cases, it had been stabbing to kill, not only to hurt. This was either professional work or that of the insane.

Over fifteen died that day and many more the next week, almost from every religion, but with one common thread: they were all poor. The hospital turned into a large mourning station those days. Mothers and sisters, sons and daughters, brothers and wives, young and old of all religions mourned in shock while there were calls of religious harmony by the leaders, surrounded by bodyguards from their gilded bungalows.

The TV kept on shouting, 'All leaves of all the doctors and hospital staff are cancelled. Doctors not reporting immediately to work will be suspended. Negligence will not be tolerated. All hospitals have been ordered by the government to deal with the situation adequately. Necessary funds are being generated through donations. Leaders of our country have expressed shock and pain. More blood is required. They have appealed the public to donate blood.' No talk of the responsibility, of the perpetrators, or of the criminals. No talk of unprepared and severely deficient health services and severe shortage of medicines, equipment, manpower, ambulances, everything. There was no disaster management protocol.

The ward boys and *mausis* (female helpers) who cleaned the blood on the casualty floor were unusually silent for weeks later; many lost weight.

The sane in the society—the middle and lower classes, as always—lent their shoulders to the situation. People helped victims reach the hospital, bought them medicines and food, called their families, and donated money, clothes, and blood. They carried the dead bodies for funerals with the shocked families from every religion.

We all were aggrieved beyond repair, for a lifetime, for we had seen a face of our society that stays hidden—right in our backyards, ever ready to pop up again at the wish of the powerful. In the future I met many doctors from different parts of India, and they all have scars of various religious and other riots, bleeding scars that refuse to heal.

Months later, the two surgeons from two warring religions, who were in the OT in those horrible days, were in the casualty late, having tea with us all. Dr PTJ asked Dr AM, 'How's your cute son?'

Dr AM was in tears. He replied, 'I hit my son today for the first time. He was crying for a toy gun after seeing a hit movie where the hero shoots point-blank, cuts the enemy's head, stabs their tummies through and through, and blood spurts out. He wanted to do that too. There are a million laws against love and sex in this country but none against gruesome violence or killing on the screen, which stimulates kids. We proudly say India never attacked any other country but forget that we have many internally violent, warring, illiterate, and poor factions in our society, where a common man is never secure.'

He left India in a year.

CHAPTER 19

THE MOST HORRIBLE DAYS AS A DOCTOR: PART II

At about four thirty one morning, I stood with my father on the railway station platform at Nanded to receive one of his friends. The train had started from its prior station and could enter any minute now.

A familiar rumble started, and we expectedly looked afar in the dark direction of the train's arrival. There was no engine headlight visible. The rumble intensified, then we felt the tremors beneath us. Suddenly there was a crashing noise; the big glass door of the waiting room behind us shattered open, and I could see the rain of its broken shards falling upon an exodus of a panicked crowd woken up with the shouts of 'Earthquake, run!' The train had simultaneously arrived. There was an announcement to vacate the station. We received our guest and found our way out in a frightened chaos upon a shaking ground.

Next morning at the hospital, I went to the canteen for my regular tea. My colleagues were all abuzz with the news: that the earthquake that morning had killed thousands in a nearby town of Killari and surrounding areas. The aftershocks still continued, and more quakes were predicted. By noon, there was a notice in the casualty: volunteers were required to go to the site 'on personal risk' and help out with the crisis. I ran to the dean's office.

'But you married only recently . . . did you ask your wife?' the dean asked.
'I will ask her, sir,' I said.

'Okay then, report at 4 p.m. to leave,' he said gravely.

This was way before the cell phone era. There was to be no contact with family till I returned from the site.

Rushing home, I told my wife and mom. Mom, as always, was extremely upset, and told me I couldn't go unless my father agreed. He was the principal of a college and was in a meeting. I went there, called him out, and sought his permission. It was his own trait to stand up first to help when required, but this time, his voice was heavy and eyes wet. He forced himself to say yes. I touched his feet and left when he said, 'Take care, stay safe, and come back soon.'

As I returned with my knapsack and medical kit, two lists of six members each were displayed in the casualty, signed by the dean. I was to captain Team B. We were given kits for emergency treatments. We all reviewed the equipments, IV fluids, medicines, syringes, needles, etc., and started in two ambulances. It rained heavily all the way, and we reached late in the night at the local hospital building. This was the coordination centre, a few miles away from the epicentre. We were to enter the destruction zone after 5 a.m., as the electricity had failed and roads were dangerous in that rain. Sleepless, we kept on feeling the rumbling tremors and the sound like muffled lightning under the ground. It was scarier than the loudest lightning in the skies. Things kept on shaking: water in the bottles, clothes, open windowpanes, and even our hearts. We started at 5 a.m. and decided to work at different spots in pairs. Dr VB, an orthopaedic surgeon, was my partner.

In a few minutes, we entered a living hell. There were cries of pain, agony, bereavement, and psychosis. There were dead bodies everywhere; everything around us was toppled, broken, or shattered—people worst of all. As we got down at our spot with our kits, we saw the mayhem unleashed by nature and ill fate upon the people around us. Shocked relatives sat by their dead kith and kin, eyes dried, holding their heads.

There were dozens of such groups where we got down. Just as we moved a table and chair from a broken house to arrange medicines beneath a huge tree near the main road, a midsized truck stopped by. A hefty bloodstained man got down crying, shouting, using fowl language at an unknown enemy. He opened the rear compartment by lowering the plank that covers it, and we saw haphazard piles of dead bodies. He started lifting up the unclaimed, unguarded dead bodies, piling them in his truck. There was a fresh clamour of wails, and some went after him to request to take their dead for performing the last rites. He didn't deny; he asked them to pile up. Himself crying, he cursed in unthinkable language those mourning, asking them to get up and get on, that this was the wish of fate, and that those alive were in fact unlucky to have survived.

We started searching for the injured and found them everywhere. Helping them sit or lie down, giving them antibiotics and painkillers, bandaging their wounds, starting IV fluids in the dehydrated, immobilizing their fractured, twisted limbs, and moving them to temporary shelters occupied us for a few hours.

Those with bleeding wounds, head injuries, fractures, and those who were unconscious were moved beneath a tree near the main road, where ambulances could pick them up on their way to the coordination centre. A volunteer started recording their vitals.

There were many volunteers from many organisations, most of them common men and women. The Indian military was heading the operations. I have never seen more organised and selfless extreme hard work. Some volunteers distributed water bottles thankfully.

As most of the houses were made of stones and wooden logs, the death and injury toll was massive. We were still feeling the shocks beneath us and were advised to stay away from dilapidated structures.

At about 3 p.m., we were fatigued mentally in the face of death. There was nowhere we could look and not find dead bodies or mourners. This trauma affected both me and VB at almost the same time, and we sat upon out table and cried silently for a few minutes, when someone asked if we wanted to have food. Food? Here? Who will want to eat?

But the human body is way beyond mental control unless you are a practising saint. We realised we were really hungry and weak, and if we wanted to help others further, we had to be strong and healthy.

A religious group had made a tent where volunteer ladies cooked meals, and those in relief work were being invited and served. For the victims, there were packets being distributed wherever they were. We washed hands and went in. There, at 5 p.m., we ate our food in the name of God, sitting guiltily in a tent surrounded by dead bodies and wails only a few feet away. I always shiver at the memory.

This followed for three days after that, as we travelled into the deep interiors, watching the manic destruction that nature can inflict. There were many things worth wondering.

There was a village where all the people, from infants to the elderly, made a group early morning and sang hymns/bhajans praising the lord. Almost everyone who could walk even with support came out. Almost everyone from this entire village survived the earthquake. A few of those at home suffered injuries.

A whole family was woken up by hissing of a large cobra and ran out of the house, surviving the quake that happened just then.

The ground at the epicentre, a place called Ekondi Lohara, actually appeared tilted. The electric poles leaned, angulated to the ground, broken wires hanging from them. A farmer who had witnessed the actual quake, having woken up for travelling, told us that he felt as if the ground was a quivering leaf in a tornado. He said he actually saw the crops and poles tilted almost horizontal.

There was a very tall wall; the three floors of the house it had supported had collapsed, and one could see the dusty, destroyed interior. At the top was a window, a bed beside it on the half portion of the remaining floor and a leg hanging down that bed. It was the richest farmer in that village who could keep an eye upon his land from that window. They couldn't reach up there in time to save him, so he was left alone there, awaiting a crane to arrive in a day or two.

We also witnessed a pair of parrots that were rescued alive from a house in which there were no survivors. The strong cage had kept the birds alive. People were found dead in all positions, mostly in their sleep, unaware of what befell them.

From the third day onwards, there was utter chaos, anarchy, and riots of immorality. As the survivors begged for food and clothes, running after every vehicle they saw, risking the lives of their children and themselves to get food, there were fights among them.

Some people dug the collapsed debris, searching for gold over dead bodies and in their homes, money, ornaments, etc. The military men caught many people at it, dealing severely with them. Some posed as administrators or grieving relatives, conning donations from innocent donors who suffered a shock of sympathy. Some took advantage of the foreigners who had brought with them good quality of clothes, equipment, and other stuff. I even remember how we humiliated and boycotted a junior doctor who had stolen a costly Littmann stethoscope from an aid centre of a foreign NGO, until he returned it. Media was fairly responsible then and helped people reach out to their families.

An ocean of humanity oozed out too. Many warring religious organisations and factions who would otherwise never come to a negotiation table worked together in this crisis without any guidance. India unites in the face of crisis like a fanatic family, far wider than the cricket or entertainment community.

I remember the massive tents by the Bank of Maharashtra (I think the Jalna branch), which served hot food and cold water in a farm, sending vans to all nearby areas to bring relief workers and drop them back after feeding them. Someone gave us blankets too.

Then the heavy rains started. Wet, decomposing dead bodies raised a massive stink, and there were traffic jams due to mismanaged crowds. Everyone wanted to help; there was no mechanism to control the swarms of people and vehicles entering the narrow roads that had many blocks.

Our team had exhausted its supplies, and survivors who could be helped were mostly all shifted to the makeshift hospitals. There were innumerable stories of lost families, lone survivors, and so many shades of grief and bereavement. In five minutes, nature had killed or wounded thousands, orphaned many, destroyed billions' worth of property and crops, shocked the world, and revealed the naked, shameful truth: nobody was prepared. There was no disaster management cell anywhere then.

As we returned to the town where we bedded, we heard the appeals of donation in cash by various leaders. In a country where many were listed among the Forbes billionaires and many leaders owned thousands of acres of land and massive properties, there were appeals to the general population for cash to help victims of a natural disaster. Many business houses, organisations, and individuals came forward, who adopted villages to be recreated.

After a week, we planned to return, and I could make a call to my home from the coordination centre, telling them that I was returning the next day.

We all returned as changed people. Whenever someone boasts now of their abilities or might, I smile sadly in my mind. That week taught us how futile, fragile, and unpredictable life is and how helpless humans are. It also showed us the many ways in which one can contribute to the world and the importance of being prepared. The cloud of that mass devastation of life had only one silver lining: we were all proud to be able to stand up first in the face of that crisis.

As I entered my home next evening, I found my father waiting in the front porch in his trademark white pyjamas, sitting cross-legged on his favourite chair.

Also with his trademark pride for his son.

CHAPTER 20

THE SUFFERING AFTER DEATH

A friend's wife was once admitted with severe burns. She had caught fire while cooking alone at home.

After admitting her at a government hospital where I was a student, my devastated friend called me for help. Their whole family was in a wordless shock. The couple had married a year earlier. The doctors had calculated the percentage of burns and predicted a very poor chance of survival. My friend was dead scared of it all. His only relief was that she had clearly stated in her dying declaration that she was alone at home and it was by mistake that her sari had caught fire. She categorically mentioned to the police and doctors that her husband had treated her with utmost love and it was her own mistake that led to this accident.

She passed away in three days. Till then, my friend sat on the stairs near the burns ward, clutching his head, moving only to have tea or visit washrooms. She was shifted to the mortuary for post-mortem examination, mandatory in every medico-legal case.

The drama began.

In a usual post-mortem examination, after the external examination of the dead body is complete, the skull, chest, and abdomen are cut open by instruments. After removing samples from stomach, intestines, and small pieces of some internal organs, the body is sewn back with needles and thread.

The mortuary attendant, frankly stinking of country liquor, called my friend in and told him the rates of 'routine' versus 'special' treatment of the body in artificially sympathetic words that hurt more than any other. The routine would mean haphazard, unclean cutting open, while the special included clean cuts. The suturing back after the post mortem exam could be done routinely like everyone else, or specially, with care, to look better so that the sutures were hidden. For a special treatment, more money would be required. I told my friend that I would tell my professors and have the attendant punished, but he declined. He was mature and knew the ways of the world.

'Take good care of her. Don't hurt her too much,' he said, while handing over the money without any questions. The first attendant went in. A second one came out.

'Shall I use the old bed sheet to cover her up after the post-mortem, or do you have a new one?' asked the second one.

He took some more money to get a new bed sheet.

As we awaited a provisional death certificate to take her for cremation, a man came to us from outside the mortuary. 'Do you have a hearse already or do you need one? Because I am leaving now—my duty is over. You will have to arrange outside campus.' It was 6 p.m. already. We asked him what he would charge. His answer, as expected, was ten times higher than a taxi car would charge a passenger. As he said, there was no option.

My friend's family, all mourning, stood outside the mortuary, where there was no place or shade for any relatives to sit or stand. Many shocked and inconsolable relatives wailed in groups; some collapsed. Some stunned faces stared at the sky, while others stared at the ground.

We took the body and left.

As we entered the cremation site, a few young and old men actually caught hold of our hands, pulling us in different directions, claiming that they were the official, the best, etc.

After we showed the certificate for the permission for cremation, we were allowed to take the body inside. There followed a rate chart of wood quality and quantity, and every other commodity required to perform the rites, small and big, from flowers to rice, rated far above any market. The marketing strategy was universally the same: 'Do you want best for your dead or low quality?'

The stunned family went on distributing money to one and all who asked for it. Here, at the last place one can visit upon the earth, there was no concern either for life or for humanity.

After many customs and rituals, the fire rose to offer the final mercy to her body.

Just as the fresh bouts of agonised cries shattering the skies sank into heart-wrenching sobs of many, my friend, who till now had kept his woe frozen, started crying openly, looking at the pyre.

Someone approached him again, stinking of cheap liquor and much more.

'Sir, I will protect the pyre overnight and collect the bones tomorrow morning, if you want. Otherwise dogs, cats, or birds eat them up,' he said. 'But you will have to pay me all the money now.' (Ashes/bones were to be immersed in the River Ganges after the cremation.) He took his share.

He was nowhere to be seen next morning, but he had collected the bones and left them with his friend, who said we had to wait till the 'bone collector' returned because he didn't know what the deal was or if the money had already been paid. After we paid him too, my friend collected the remains and returned.

When there is a big wound, smaller wounds do not hurt.

While most of the traditions are respectable and meaningful, the commercial execution of these today needs to evolve. Better understanding of the mourning family and friends at all these stages will go a long way in lessening their sufferings.

SECTION II

THE DOCTOR

CHAPTER 21

MEDICAL ANGELS I MET UPON EARTH: PART I

KEM Hospital Mumbai
Ward 10
2.30 p.m., somewhere in 1999

Dr Sorab Bhabha, neurologist, entered the clinic room.

Dr RNR, my seniormost chief resident appearing for DM neurology exams, was to present a case to him. Three other batches of DM students, almost twenty others including medicine residents, lecturers, and interns had gathered in that small room, strategically located to see all but hide faces to duck direct questioning. The patient sat on the couch, a case of ADEM (acute disseminated encephalomyelitis).

Dr Bhabha took his chair in the centre. Suave. A face that oozed brilliance and kindness, only balanced by the mockery in his eyes. A smile that was a punchline before anyone even started. Very fair, thin-built. Cream and brown dress, dark tie. English in appearance. Camel-skin knapsack, reddish-brown shoes. Stubble and carelessly tossed back hair. All in all, the picture-perfect genius.

Of course, Dr RNR, however studied he was, was trembling. There is nothing academically more enjoyable for medical PG students than the case presentation by a senior who they know is going to be skinned and scarred alive. It's a dessert. RNR started.

What followed was two hours of a dream. We forgot where we were, we got lost into his descriptive interpretation, analysis, and differential. He actually created a vision of the entire visual pathway there in the centre of the room, only with his words, hand movements, and eyes. When he concluded the differential, we knew we were with one of the topmost neurological minds in the world. There couldn't have been other possibilities. He had 'caged' the case. Boldly, people asked him questions, and smiling, he answered. Point-and-shoot answers.

Of course he didn't entirely disappoint us on the skinning front. 'Hammer ka awwaaz toh bahut aa raha hai, Professor, reflex nahi aa raha' meaning 'Your hammer makes a lot of noise, but one can't yet see the reflex', etc. The only difference was that the one being skinned also laughed at the crisp, stinging, tacit sarcasm for its accuracy and the unmatched beauty of his language.

Upon finishing the tutorial clinic, he started to walk his fast cadence towards the parking. I ran and asked him about a complicated case that we could not understand, and my other teachers had suggested I discuss the case with him too (old man, confused and convulsing three days without fever/stroke/trauma/infection/metabolic abnormality or prior history). He asked me to summarise the history and clinical examination in minimum words. As I did, he said 'Google *serotonin syndrome*.' I did. The patient went home in a few days, completely improved. The connection of this syndrome and the drugs that the patient took was published only recently.

Whatever we asked, he made it a point to explain from the very basic. He was very compassionate to everyone but intolerant of any hypocrisy, show, or lying. He didn't spend time arguing where it was a waste of time. 'I have worked upon five continents, rajas, and the best clinical experience one can acquire is in India. Don't waste any time in arguing with anyone, however small or big. Mention your point twice, smile, and leave.' God! How much that has always helped me!

Once, a kid with stimulus-sensitive epilepsy was being presented. Upon patting the shoulder of this five-year-old girl, she would go in a flurry of what appeared to be myoclonic/jerky movements, only a tad prolonged (maybe a second longer). We all were eliciting it to present it to him and trying our own analyses of what was happening.

In he came. Case started. As the presenter raised his hand to demonstrate, Dr Bhabha said no. We all were so eager to show him what happens when the child was tapped. Cell phone videos were not yet available. But he declined. 'None of us has the right to precipitate a seizure, even if for learning. It is discomfort for the patient,' he said.

I have rarely seen that kind of affection for a patient again.

Eventually my turn came to present a case. Anxiety peaked, and my ego started quivering like a jelly. The happy gathering was all curious to see the new resident (yours truly) being painted black and blue. I started the history after basic data: 'Sir, the patient had some gluteal intramuscular injection and, within a few minutes, had blebs and rashes only on that leg then became paralysed in that leg then in the other after a few hours.'

'Dear Professor [that was his pet sarcastic name for any new resident doctor], just because someone sitting by a moonlit pond had a seizure, you don't call it *lunarogenic epilepsy!*'

I willingly joined everyone in the laughter that followed. I had my ego too, and it revolted. After the case was over, I went to the patient, who was still admitted in the same ward, and asked him about the correctness of history. Once he confirmed, I ran back and, trembling, asked Dr Bhabha, 'Sir, I apologise, but I confirmed with the patient, and he assures that it was so. Would you like to confirm?'

He smiled. 'If you're sure you are correct, never apologise. Truth will show itself. Now find out what that injection could have been.'

My fear of him disappeared, and respect multiplied. I stalked him and followed everything he said.

(Will continue as part II.)

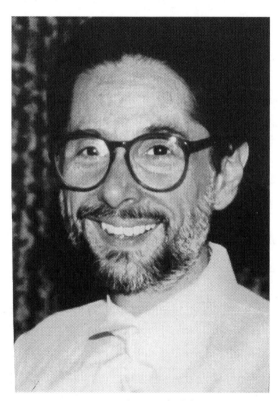

Dr Sorab K. Bhabha

CHAPTER 22

MEDICAL ANGELS I MET UPON EARTH: PART II

Due to some administrative glitches, Dr Sorab Bhabha left KEM Hospital, Mumbai.

He still visited us at KEM for the famous neuro-radiology meet on Fridays at 8 a.m. This was the war zone of titans, and we learnt the meaning of 'academically cruelly perfect' in that room. They all screwed us together, but we were, anyway, insignificant 'chillupillus' in that room; they also skinned each other to dissect the truth. References were called for, textbooks were opened, and whoever bled, truth prevailed! We grew up as a doctor each such Friday. This was the ultimate in our academics then, because Mumbai's stalwart specialists took the first row while the resident docs from neurology, radiology, medicine, orthopaedics, and paediatrics presented the cases to discuss MRI/CT scans/X-rays, etc.

Once someone questioned Dr Bhabha's comment about the blood supply of medial pons. He smiled mockingly, said he knew he was right. They called in a textbook. He looked at us, not in the textbook. As he smiled at us students, he said with his trademark wink, 'Let them search. I know.' He was, of course, correct, and I still remember some sourly bitter faces.

Intellectual fights between different medical specialties are legendary, and the physician–surgeon cold wars are well established. Dr Bhabha's humour was our greatest weapon in our residency for this cause. 'Don't talk like lumpologists, bumpologists, carpenters, or plumbers,' he'd say when we made a mistake in differential analysis, and we shamelessly enjoyed it (along with the lumpologists, etc. who accompanied us)! But he was very good friends with most surgeons, and they made fun of him too ('By the time you neuros evaluate one patient, we can finish a conference').

Only once did he intellectually assault one of the senior orthopaedic surgeons who had crossed his own boss (this ortho boss had advised against surgery) in an attempt to be (over)smart. His assault was the sweetest, most polite series of questions that led the presenting 'smarty' into his own trap. 'So when you say you examined the patient and found he had absolutely normal neurological examination, did you feel the need, Doctor, to obtain another opinion from a trained neurologist, especially because the patient was having symptoms without signs? An exceptionally highly educated and skilled doctor like yourself must have surely thought why the patient had pain and disabling weakness with a normal examination, and if the patient worsened after surgery, did you feel the need to connect these two coincidences, to cross-examine yourself?'

I haven't seen more sweat on a single doctor since then!

As he didn't come to KEM any more, I started to go to Hinduja Hospital at Mahim to attend his OPD. I wrote notes; he dictated upon the case sheets. I was slightly proud of writing good notes in readable handwriting and then showing him in anticipation of some praise from my idol. It came only once. He asked me if I remembered the patient we were seeing in OPD. I replied that I hadn't seen that patient earlier. He smiled and said, 'See his old file—you will see the beautiful handwriting of a doctor with memory loss!'

* * *

'I have been diagnosed with motor neurone disease.' Dr Bhabha told me on a rainy day in his Hinduja OPD. 'You should not think about this, try and concentrate upon your exams'.

I couldn't even cry. Having lost my father a few months earlier, I was still depressed.

'There are very few years left, and I am winding up' He told as officially as one can.

After a few minutes he dictated someone on phone a complete recipe of a delicious Parsi dish, and joked about how one can spoil it with a small mistake. Patients in the OPD on that day too all went home happy and satisfied as always. I never saw a tear in his eyes, but an eternity was sobbing in his courageous smile.

He never asked or accepted any favour from any student. He never talked to please someone, but was never rude. He never ever showed his weaknesses or pain to anyone.

Dr Anand Alurkar was his favourite student too, and I secretly envied Anand who had so many of Dr Bhabha's qualities himself. He liked Anand's case presentations. They both understood the crying necessity of the parsimony of words while engaging in academic discussions, a rare quality among intellectuals. Otherwise, most academic discussions are like a marketplace of intellectuals who almost get violent to show off unnecessary stored knowledge, often out of context.

Dr Bhabha taught me that even conversion reaction (where the patient feels that he/she has an illness and deeply believes it in spite of not having it), malingering (where patient knows he/she is not sick but pretends so), functional (same as malingering, or exaggerating true illness), irritating (imagine your professional rival) patients need good care, understanding, and compassion. One should never look down upon them as a waste of time.

One day I asked him something about spinal cord infarctions. After speaking a few minutes about it, he went into a trance. 'You must strive to be the best in your chosen field, not to show off or achieve, just to feel the pleasure of it. Learn the most standard, not the shortcuts. There will be slower people, people who enjoy repetition and routine for decades . . . you need to keep up to your own speed, not theirs. If you can do something faster, do it, but without compromising upon its quality. Don't speak or explain—just do it. When someone thinks about your work, it should be gold standard for that time, if not better.'

On the eve that my results for DM neuro exams in Mumbai University were out, he called me at his home at Cuffe Parade. A rosewood interior in a huge bungalow, a large white piano, and a great Dane welcomed me around him.

His smile was my pride in that moment. 'Congratulations!' He beamed. 'You should be proud, Mr Topper!'

'Don't think about those who talk about you, good or bad. People sideline themselves eventually to their destination. You must continue to walk to yours. And what people say is *not* your destination,' he said once.

Selected for a Canadian fellowship, I made up my mind *not* to go, as I had already been away from wife and kids for three years by then for my DM course. Another real reason, 'no money', was too embarrassing to admit. When I called him, he said, 'Close your eyes, do what it takes, and go without a second thought just because I say so.'

That one 'order' has changed my life.

He made my CV himself ('*Woh tera* biography change *karr* . . . make it human and decent'). He told me that family is the greatest distraction in research, so I had to make my decisions carefully. I still took my family with me and realised that I could have done better without distraction. Truth is very heavy and unpleasant. But it was also him who had advised me, 'Whatever decisions you make, involve your family, for in the end they are the only ones who stay with you and matter.'

I saw him last just before boarding my Toronto flight. He sat like Buddha, smiling, knowing I may cry any time.

'New shoes *haan*? Very essential for research!' he said as I struggled not to weaken.

'I bought shoes just like yours, sir,' I said.

'I know you are scared of flying. But this is a good airline, and mostly, nothing happens. Take good care. Winters are quite bad there. And eat well. Don't spend like a king there.'

'Sir, I want a picture of yours,' I said.

His smile waned a bit, then he said, 'Yes, my wife will give it to you, but don't do its puja, okay?' And he beamed again!

'Sir, I will come back and meet you in two years.'

'Yes, we will meet.'

I touched his feet. That was to be the last time I saw him.

I called him every week from London ON. He guided me and supported and nurtured my strengths, while understanding my weaknesses. 'Everyone has their own weaknesses, and it's okay. Don't feel guilty for your weaknesses or fears.'

Once there was a crisis, and I quit one fellowship because of humiliating behaviour of one boss. The UWO (God bless them) actually acted against that boss and offered me another fellowship, but I was required to clear another viva exam and furnish a recommendation letter. I cleared the viva. Dr Bhabha stood by my morale, helped me overcome this crisis, wrote the required recommendation to the UWO, and I got my fellowship.

In his last conversation, he asked me if I wished my old boss at the hospital (the one I had quit) if we happened to cross each other's path. I said I earlier had but had stopped as the OB didn't reply. He told me, 'Never let that happen. Smile and wish, even if he does not reply. A smile can convey almost everything you actually want to say. *Who* is not important. *What* is right is important.'

Then he asked me what I actually ate, if I slept well, and how my family was and told me to concentrate upon intensive care and IPD patients too.

'We will meet. I am waiting for you to return,' he reassured me when he sensed I was crying.

Then I received the email of his passing away at the young age of fifty-two.

His shadow has, ever since, guided me. He still laughs at me if any lies, any compromises, any hypocrisy is inevitable for me. 'You can live without these,' he winks and says. In every patient, every dilemma, every complication, his approach helps me sail through. Now I know what he meant when he said, 'We will meet.' He has kept his promise!

My greatest certificate in life yet is his 'queen square hammer', which his wife, Dr Firoza Bhabha, graciously passed on to me as his blessing.

If you need people for being strong, you are a mob.

If you can stand alone strong, you are a man.

Dr Sorab K. Bhabha taught me how to be a man: both in medicine and in life.

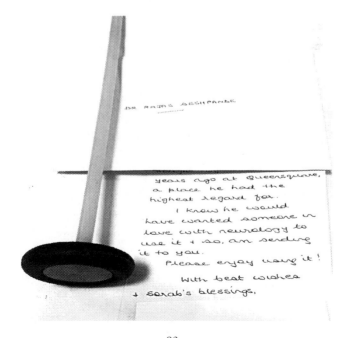

CHAPTER 23

MEDICAL ANGELS I MET UPON EARTH: PART III

'My decision is final. You can kill me now,' said my professor to the mob in his room, about twenty hardcore muscular giants in the trademark outfit of a dreaded political party.

He was just about five feet and thin built and sat placidly upon the chair in his chamber. I stood behind the mob, terrified, vaguely wondering what would be the best self-defence and escape in that small old homely room. There also was immense anger and respect for that professor—why is he risking his life?

A political leader was arrested, this time for murder, but allegedly had many past rapes, murders, etc. to his criminal record. It is an established politico-legal tradition to develop chest pain and go to the hospital if you have enough power. Jail is only for the financially or politically poor. So this leader came to GMC Aurangabad (Ghati) Hospital with chest pain on the day of arrest by police.

I was on call. I informed my professor. He told me to completely examine the patient, do an ECG, run some blood tests, and get back to him on phone. With everything normal, he ordered overnight observation of the patient and repeat ECG next morning. That too was normal. He came for rounds. He went straight to this patient and, after examination, told the leader he was being discharged as all was well with his health.

Then came a request wrapped in an order-cum-threat: 'Don-teen divas ithech theva sahib . . . mala bara watat nahiye [Keep me admitted for two to three days more. I don't feel good].'

'Discharge him now! Then join the rounds,' the professor told me in front of the patient and moved on.

Within a few minutes, many SUVs and trucks entered the hospital. There were slogans in the name of that leader, and amidst all this, we walked with our professor to his cabin.

One good thing about a mob of goons is that they are not very articulate. They don't waste time in the service of literature. They are short and direct in their talk.

'We will kill you right here, right now, if our leader is discharged from hospital,' said the mob boss.

Medicine professor Dr Vitthal Gopalrao Kale answered the mob, 'My decision is final. You can kill me now.'

Some two to three goons actually got up, unable to think beyond obvious word meanings. Their leader asked them to hold on. Swallowing twice then with folded hands and mellowed voice, the mob boss said, 'Vichar kara, sir [think again].'

Sir didn't answer.

The mob left after few minutes of gaze-holding war.

When the police jeeps took the criminal out that day with heavy bundobust, we resident doctors felt a sense of security we had never felt before—we had a lion for our professor!

Dr VGK had mastered such situations long before any of those goons were born. He had faced morchas, verbal and physical attacks, allegations, and enquiries fearlessly. For he was the don of honesty and discipline. He stood by his words, his commitments, and principles, defending them with his life.

Joining the MD medicine course at GMC Aurangabad was associated with various anxieties and fears: genius-class teachers like Dr V. G. Kale, Dr P. Y. Muley, Dr S. G. Kulkarni, Dr D. V. Muley, Dr Mangala Borkar, Dr S. H. Talib, and Dr Anilkumar Gaikwad were all known to teach best and expect best of hard work too, but the fear of facing Dr V. G. Kale exceeded all other fears and anxieties.

* * *

No guns, no whistles, no sirens, no police in sight, but every morning at 0845 hours sharp, a curfew prevailed between the Department of Medicine office and Ward 8/9, Dr VGK's unit. Patients were in their bed, no extra relatives around, nursing staff in attention, wards cleaner than any other government premise I have ever seen, and poor resident doctors like myself with a big lump of fear in their throats hiding behind the senior residents, who mostly had the resolve and disposition of one walking towards the end of life.

He taught us the art of good medical practice.

For medicine is not only diagnosis. It is not only compassion or sweet talk. It is not only knowledge. In addition to all these, medicine is about extreme discipline, and extreme concentration, a sturdy confidence that banks only upon truth and honesty and, above all, tremendous hard work.

And that is where most of the world always locked horns with Dr V. G. Kale. He did not tolerate hanky-panky in medicine.

Ask the professor whom he threw out of the ward for not wearing an apron. Ask the nursing in-charge who faced his ire. Ask the ward boys who were transferred out, and ask hundreds of medicine residents like myself who actually stammered and trembled presenting cases to him. Say anything else they may about him—he was true, honest, and strict to the core.

'Someone's life is dependent upon what you do and how you do it,' he carved upon our hearts.

As the rounds started, a parade of clinical accuracy and truth ensued. No one could bluff him; he probably had a hidden bluff sensor.

* * *

'What is his urine sugar level today?' he asked about a chronic diabetic.

'Sir, 2 plus,' Satish, the resident doc, bluffed confidently.

'Did the doctor check your urine today?' he asked the patient.

'I didn't pass urine yet,' said the patient.

'Then this doctor must have entered your bladder while you were asleep,' he said, looking at the resident.

'Sorry, sir, it was about another patient,' Satish said. (Such medical escapes are standard in the overworked learning phase.)

'Doctor, learn to own up your mistake. If you commit a mistake and own it up, I will scold you but will still believe you. If you lie even once about a patient, I'll lose faith in you forever,' he said.

* * *

My first case presentation to him. No sleep out of fear. This patient was a sixty-five-year old with gradually increasing weakness on left half of body. I had done what I knew of the clinical examination, skipping what I thought was irrelevant. Thirty minutes before I was to present, as I came out of the washroom for the third time that morning, Dr Majid, my courteous senior, came to me in a hurry and whispered in my ear, 'Did you examine patient's scrotum?' I said no—what had it to do with paralysis on one half of body?

'Go check fast . . . and don't tell VGK that I told you.'

Patient had a mass in the scrotum, a testicular malignancy.

I took the patient for presentation.

'When did you find out about his testes?' Dr VGK asked me towards the end.

'Sir, today morning. Sorry, sir, I missed it yesterday.'

He laughed. He looked at his colleagues proudly. 'They will only learn if they are afraid of you,' he said.

* * *

An old man was sleeping with a cover upon his head during rounds, in spite of being told that Dr VGK was to see him in a few minutes. An irritated resident doctor who had been up all night and was eager to finish the rounds pulled the patient's cover sheet down when we reached him.

'Tumchya baapala pan asech uthavita kaay?' (Do you wake your father up like this?) snapped Dr VGK. We never woke up a patient again for any rounds, and if we had to, only too carefully, apologizing for the same. One sentence forever led to a change in the behaviour of ten doctors and staff on round that day.

* * *

I received a firing many times too, but the one I remember is for not supervising an intern while she was inserting needle in a patient's vein. I was nearby with another patient, and the intern poked the patient many times in an attempt to get the vein. 'Will you poke your mother so many times?' he asked us. He told us how essential it is for the doctor to feel the pain and never take the patients for granted, poor or rich, expressive or silent, good- or bad-behaved.

* * *

His elder brother, whom he respected like his father (I heard Dr VGK's voice emotional only in front of his elder brother), was admitted in our ward. Dr VGK came and asked me to collect his brother's blood for some test. With Dr VGK standing near me, when I held the syringe, my hands trembled for the first and last time in life. He took the syringe from me, collected blood in the first prick, and said, 'Your compassions, respect, or fear should never interfere with the quality of medical care.'

* * *

In today's net-based knowledge age, where students can recite the rarest of the rare syndromes but cannot examine a patient correctly, the relevance of this 'respectful fear' stands out. However Western we may become, we must face the truth: that fear (of humiliation, of verbal thrashing, of insults and sarcasm, and nothing else) alone drives most students to learn to do things accurately. Unsupervised freedom in learning life sciences quickly converts into a talkative arrogance that may turn dangerous and cost lives in medicine. This nightmare is unfolding right now and not only in India.

A police constable was sleeping, sitting upon a chair, with his rifle held between his legs, supposed to guard an admitted prisoner. Dr VGK woke him up with a sturdy pat upon his back. He thrashed the constable verbally. He started arguing arrogantly with Dr VGK and said, '*Zara Godi Gulabi ne saanga na.*' Why don't you say it with sweet words?

Dr VGK paused with his classic fierce gaze and commented, '*Tu maajhi baayko nahi ahes godine saangayla . . . police constable ahes, hi duty sodun zopne gunha aahe.*' You are not my wife to tell you in sweet words. You are a police constable. You must know it is a crime to be sleeping while on this duty.

We felt Dr VGK was being irrationally angry. But in a few weeks, another prisoner ran away from a nearby ward, shooting at the constable guarding him. We learnt later that criminals have a different way of thinking and hospitals are a good potential escape opportunity for them.

When someone is strict and honest and *not* corrupt, defamation by those hurt is the inevitable price they pay. People know where it hurts most to a straight soul. Right from partiality, casteism, dictatorship, etc., many false allegations by the displeased are rampant. And small mistakes, if any, are blown out of proportion.

He does not need me to defend anything. But I must tell here that in the three years I worked under him, he was completely impartial to the patients. No resident doctor, senior doctor, or other staff was spared mistakes or negligence in patient care, irrespective of our social/religious status. His mind was wired to teach us not only the art of medicine but the highest sense of duty.

His one-liners were terrific. He had an inherent hate of interference in clinician's work by administrators (now managements). He didn't hide it.

Once a forensic professor came to the wards in administrative capacity and asked us about some patients' medicines. After he left, Sir's face contorted in a suppressed smile. '*Unko bolo* we deal with live bodies, we do care about the outcomes, unlike in his cases!'

Once, a high-court officer called him to see a judge in a guest house for a minor complaint. Dr VGK asked him, 'Do you send ministers or judges to hospitals for holding courts or meetings if the doctors have a problem?'

'I know people may not like the way I speak, but I have never taken a favour from anyone. I don't owe it to anyone to hide the truth. And even if someone is dear to me, I wouldn't lie for them.'

Anger is misinterpreted, just like love and politeness in this world. Dr VGK was short-tempered but never unjust. He always apologised if he thought he hurt someone. I know of many colleagues, teachers, who depended upon Dr Kale to speak the truth, which they couldn't. He helped many in crises, but very few stood by him in his difficult times.

Medical knowledge and skill, however advanced, have to stand upon a base made up of fearless honesty, truth, discipline of body and mind both, and concentration. A doctor without these qualities becomes a medical businessman, not a respectable doctor.

My fondest memory of Dr Kale is this: On one Teachers' Day when we resident doctors felicitated our teachers in the department of medicine, his answer to the decoration was 'If a policeman catches a thief, it is his duty. He must not expect any praise for it. It is my duty to be a good teacher, the best I know, and to make the best doctors possible out of you all. I don't need any felicitation for doing my duty. God bless you!'

Thank you, Dr V. G. Kale, sir, for teaching this to thousands of students over thirty-five years, driving but a scooter (yes, we were afraid of that green

Bajaj scooter too) and living a life of simplicity that will always be an example for us.

I am proud to have trained under a brave-hearted saint like you.

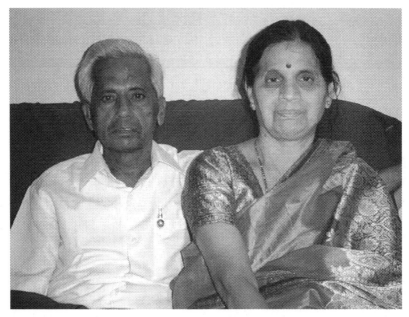

Dr V. G. Kale with Mrs Kale.

CHAPTER 24

MEDICAL ANGELS I MET UPON EARTH: PART IV

'He's a king . . . and also a superman,' Deb said.

One of the most respected figures in the world of clinical and research neurology, director of a specialty unit and professor in one of the best reputed western universities, and the highest among genius masters I had met in my life yet, Dr John Bach was also the favourite swoon of many women and some men at the university hospital.

I was dining in the only Indian restaurant in that Canadian city with Ravi and Philip from India, Deb from Australia, Maria from Canada, and Paula from Argentina. We worked in different units but heard almost daily about Dr John Bach from Deb, who was his fellow of two years, and she was oh-so much in awe of his personality.

This neurology set-up was one of the last places one could refer patients to, the top of the referral pyramid in world neurology. Giants, stalwarts, and titans were commonplace in this department. These names were familiar because we had read textbooks written by them; diseases, syndromes, and procedures were named after them, and some had become immortal by their contribution to medicine: Nobel winners and their co-workers, the creator of aneurysm clips, and the world's best in stroke, to name a few.

This was different from the Indian experience in many ways; although these people were among the topmost in the world, they still greeted you even if you were a student. You could talk frankly, have coffee, and share lunch, call them by their first name, and they would not mind standing behind you in the coffee queue. Nobody misused students to get personal work done. No high-handedness as a teacher. In short, students were treated very well, almost equal. The more dwarfed you are psychologically, the more you tend to demand respect and show people down. Very few medical seniors understood this. The only superiority most of these giants donned was their work, and that alone was sufficient to intimidate the students.

Once, while we were dining in this Indian restaurant, Dr Bach walked in. An ecstatic Deb introduced us to him.

About six feet three inches, German looks, thin but strongly built, scanty hair, restless hands and feet, with a handsome face that reminded me of Ayn Rand's words: 'the face without pain or fear or guilt!'

He finished his dinner before us and left. The waiter brought some desserts. He told us, 'Dr Bach has paid your bills. He added these desserts to your order.' Deb laughed aloud. 'I told you!' she said.

'Thank you, sir,' I said as Dr John Bach entered the OPD the next morning.

'Pleasure!' he said, as if nothing had happened to his hundred-plus dollars.

He asked, 'How fast do you do a neurophysical examination of a patient in OPD?'

'Twelve minutes,' I replied proudly. 'We are used to timing.' (A routine screening neurological examination in outpatient set-up is a minimum eighty steps and may extend beyond 120 different things a neurologist must check. Skipping any is dangerous.)

'That's too much time. I take three minutes.' He handsomely smiled.

Now this lure was irresistible.

'Sir, I would like to see for myself once.'

'Call me John, not Sir. Join me in OPD when free.'

My boss Dr JJ once humiliated me and my colleague to impress some female student, and we had an argument. This argument repeated, and to get back, he cancelled the permission he had given me to bring my wife and kids from India to stay with me. I quit.

Serendipity then did a Heimlich's upon my future.

Dr Bach asked if I wanted to join him, as Deb was leaving. If I passed the interview, I could join, with almost thrice the stipend. The day I joined Dr Bach, my world changed forever.

He did teach me his own technique of performing an OPD neurological exam in three minutes, without missing the details. He was a medical genius, for the lack of any superlative adjective. Right from the origin of medical words to the newest pharmacological advances, he had it all on the tip of his tongue.

His concentrated gaze, that genius torch of brain and eyes, was like a laser beam picking up every abnormality; registering, categorizing, analyzing, and assimilating every small and big detail; discarding the unnecessary; and reaching a conclusion just as he finished the examination. He was twice the character Sherlock Holmes to me. If he had a doubt, he innocently asked us students. Mostly we couldn't answer, then we ran with him to the computer and found the best to be offered to the patient. There was no pretending, high-handedness, or an 'I know all and better than you' attitude unlike most teachers. And no unnecessary show of knowledge by diverted discussions.

He taught me that unless you answer each question the patient wants to ask, the consult is not over, and he also taught me how to 'steer' people who keep on asking the same questions, initiate irrelevant discussion, or speak vaguely. He was as tactful as a mother would be to her child, in case bad news was to be shared with the patient.

* * *

'I have been isolated and boycotted, Rjaas [that's what he called me], by most of the international community, for speaking the truth. People do not like it. More than half the research is either misdirected, twisted, or almost useless. Huge funds cross hands to manipulate data. You can then get almost *any* reference on pubmed to prove yourself correct. At least one can generate enough confusion for his contention to be accepted.'

'Be it blind replication of western research, statistical collections, manipulating data, conducting trials rejected by the developed world as unethical or dangerous, or tweaking studies to publish them as one's own, India is also one of the largest playgrounds for such practices.'

He taught me the intricacies of research analysis.

'*Nightmare* is too insufficient a word to describe what is going on in medical research today. Studies are planned with a specific point to prove, and data is manipulated accordingly, right from the patient selection to the interpretation of outcomes. There are committees paid highly to sort out or mask the unwanted inferences. The standard double-blind placebo controlled multicentre international seal of authenticity has many holes, although there is no bypass to it. It's like democracy—in the absence of a better system, the majority supervenes, and if the majority is corrupt, there is no option but to submit.'

He showed me two documents: an original FDA drug report about a new molecule and its actually published (manipulated) version. The difference was comparable only to that between a child's mind and a murderer's. Most practising doctors, students, and patients are blinded to what happens behind the scenes of a drug's research and launch. The costlier the drug, the more the chances of professional infidelity. The vehement prescription of any new drug launched is a great threat to today's medicine.

Dr R. B. Bhagwat, one of the most senior and respected physicians in Aurangabad, India, was once examining my grandma. I was a PG medical student at Aurangabad GMC then. I had asked him his opinion about Alprazolam, a newly launched drug then. 'There is a honeymoon period for every drug,' he had said, 'your final opinion must survive that period. That 'magic' drug then is now the addiction of thousands all over the world.

Ten years later, Dr Bach thus showed me the proof of this.

'Never presume,' said Dr John Bach. 'Never take anything for granted. Question everything, right from the sanity, intention, and wisdom of one saying it, however big the other person be, whatever his post and credentials. Challenge everything' he said often! Whenever someone said 'In my experience' during an academic discussion, Dr Bach laughed aloud and said, 'You just murdered the logical science in this argument!'

He loved it if I could catch his mistakes. He rewarded me if I proved him wrong. He is the only doctor I met who, in spite of being twenty years my senior and a global big shot, once took me to other consultant friends in OPD and told them proudly that his student proved him wrong. There was no question of ever presuming I knew better . . . for he was the master, but unlike many other masters I had met, he was open to others being correct and him being wrong too. We all need to accept that some rare times students or juniors are correct, we may be wrong, and egos should not interfere with a doctor's analysis or diagnosis.

For in the field of medicine, nothing is above the good of a patient, and the doctor alone has the capacity to guard that good.

Lying to a patient is equal to double blasphemy: you kill their trust and your own integrity. One can understand exceptions like reassuring a dying patient, lying to avoid violence, and lying in a hope to calm down some patients who may harm themselves; beyond that, the margins blur.

We in India have also the concern of rampant 'illiterate, gunda culture', which is averse to truth and expects Bollywoodian doctors and events.

I had to go somewhere once and had not my own car yet. Without my saying a word, he gave me the keys to his Lexus, no questions asked. I had no dental insurance and needed a tooth out. He sent me to his dentist and paid my bills (dental services are very costly in the developed world). He always respectfully introduced me to his patients and praised me too (undeserved, I agree). He protected me from racist patients.

He played violin at concerts. He was an excellent connoisseur of wines. His reading was voracious, and his sense of humour out of the world. His English was impeccable. We played a game of using a minimum number of words to express things. He challenged me if I could shorten any of his sentences without altering their meaning. Only few like him would know how precious time is. This habit of not beating around the bush and avoiding every single unnecessary word has added years to my life.

* * *

I asked him, 'How does a practising physician or student distinguish between true and pseudo knowledge or research in medicine? If so many research trials are manipulated, what to believe?' He introduced me to the Cochrane database, which analyses claimed research outcomes, and lists the good, the bad, and also the unknown about most drugs and also taught me how to discover the hidden information within a trial. He trained me also to check the details of patients enrolled in a study. It was common observation that claims of a drug being very good in a study usually were associated with enrolment of milder cases with lesser chances of progression and better chances of recovery. Whether this was the normal course of that disease in those patients or the thousand-dollar drug really helped them was difficult to dissect.

'Rjaas, one must cut off all the glamour, lights, orchestra, aura, and the desire of social acceptance to see the naked truth about anything. The real nature of a person or something they contend can only be seen then,' he said when he gifted me the Eskimo hunting spectacles (seen below) made of seal bone, which cut off all the light reflected by the snow on all sides so one can see only the target through small slits in those spectacles. And yes, he never wrapped a gift.

We could criticise each other and make fun of the differences we had. He was German by origin and did have a bias like all of us do, based upon some of his experiences. He desperately tried to change himself here.

'Do you have these rides in India, Rjaas?' he asked when I returned from the Toronto National Fair.

'No, Dr Bach, we have different rides.' (I was too embarrassed to admit that my country was ten years behind those helicopter rides.)

'Then what do you have, tiger or elephant rides?' he sarcastically beamed.

'Yes, sir, and many Canadians come to India to enjoy them.'

We both laughed.

'I once had a psychotic fellow,' he told me. And then he laughed loudly and said, 'That fellow can also use the same sentence about me.'

He readily understood that people may dislike or isolate him for being superior, far better, and also gay. He was not sure if we Indians would accept his orientation, so he initially was reserved about it, but then he did invite us all to a party in his palatial bungalow, one of the most beautifully adorned homes I have seen, with busts of Napoleon, Aristotle, Plato, Darwin, etc. in every nook and corner.

Like the range of sound for human hearing is limited only to certain decibels, some intellectual processes, some feelings, some emotions are out of range for most, and in general, people are scared of what they don't understand. To expect an individual with average IQ to completely grasp the thought processes and behaviour of a genius is unjust and irrational. We readily end up labelling higher-placed intellect madness.

Although Dr Bach usually neglected those who did not understand him, most of the world around him was 'two sandwiches short of a picnic' for him. He did not waste time for the ill-behaved, irrational, and hypocrites.

He was always excited like a child to learn something new in neurology, and he refused to be at peace with a question mark lurking in his mind. For umpteen times a day, I ran with him seven floors up and down to discuss with a radiologist or pathologist about a case in OPD, and the patients seen by him never carried home a question mark about their medical facts.

He wore a limited edition (only sixty made) Swatch with a brain as a dial and vasculature as the hands. He told me that it was no longer sold. I naturally obtained one online in a few days (seen below). I love this watch much more because it reminds me of him every day. He also got me addicted to own the best of digital technology and to put it to use for personal and patient care.

Dr Bach gave me the two most precious academic opportunities of my life, those of writing chapters as first author in two highly reputed neurology textbooks. This crown of my CV is thanks to him. When I told him this was one of my dreams, he said, 'Well, dream the next one now, there's no time to waste.'

A day before I left Canada, Dr Bach invited me and my family for a dinner, and he cooked almost twelve dishes, half of them Indian. He did get emotional when he commented, 'Rjaas, you will have to grow up one day to the painful fact that medical achievements always fall short of expectations. I have spent twenty-six years seeing neurology patients. I had a terrific career and saved many, but my quest of finding a solution to this one disease [his specialty] always eluded me.'

I knew a part of this by experience: when you don't achieve what you set out to achieve, whatever else you achieve seems meaningless, and there is no solace to the intellect in mindless repetition of the routine.

Medical market is driven by money, also necessary for its own sustenance, research, and growth. When the majority makes decisions and the majority likes money, one can readily understand the obligations upon many decisions. We live a world where if you don't fall in line with the majority, you mostly sacrifice your social career. When researchers directly or indirectly invest in pharma shares, we don't need a trial to predict the outcome! I was surprised to the core when at an international conference at Vienna, he told me in advance about some speakers who would speak/camp for a particular medicine.

The tears in Dr Bach's eyes that day represented the agony of hundreds of medical practitioners and researchers all over the world who want to live an honest and glorious life of achievements but whose dreams are sabotaged by their own medical community, governments, and a society near-totally blinded to the truth of what goes on in medical research.

Today there are achievers, but there could have been ten in place of one. There is good research, but only a tiny percentage, and the divine class of medical geniuses who set out to change the world by finding cures and solutions is dying every passing day, to be replaced by profit-based practices and research.

Dr Bach changed me completely, purified my soul, and taught the most important thing of all: to proudly accept who I am, to pursue what my intellectual self demands of me with passion, love, dedication, and the intensity of one who understands how short and unpredictable life is!

He thus added the remaining two sandwiches to the wonderful picnic of my life.

PS:

Name changed. Dr John Bach is an imaginary name.

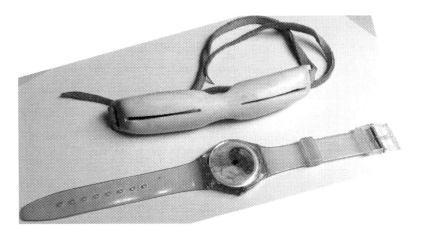

CHAPTER 25

MEDICAL ANGELS I MET UPON EARTH: PART V

Some patients taught me a lot about life. Here's how:

The breathless grandpa.

This octogenarian Mr Abaji was admitted for the umpteenth time in the general ward for sudden breathlessness due to a respiratory condition called COPD. In the general ward at government hospitals, there's barely three feet distance between beds, without any privacy (not even curtains between beds). On the first day, the old patient on Mr Abaji's right side passed away. In a few hours, the young one on his left also became critical, had to be intubated, and was kept on artificial breathing through a rubber bag called an ambu bag. Resident doctors and relatives took turns 24/7 to keep on pressing the ambu bag fourteen times a minute till the ICU ventilators became available. (There were only two ventilators for twenty wards; each ward had forty patients.)

Mr Abaji usually always smiled, but death four feet away on one side and another in waiting on the other side had dampened his smile. Still breathless at 2 a.m., he called me, smiled, and said, 'Aamchi baari anik ekda chukli dacter.' Look, they missed my turn again!

He told me next, 'Save him first, Doctor. I have seen life. He is young. I will pray God to take me away instead of him.' Then he did fold his hands and actually prayed.

He had no relatives.

What with his prayers and my professor's treatment, both of them went home well.

* * *

The Illiterate Gold Heart

This huge man of about fifty-five years, an illiterate farmer from Rajasthan who always wore a bright yellow turban, was suspected to have liver cancer. My boss told me to proceed with a liver biopsy. Although I had assisted my senior resident to do it, I had not done it myself, and the senior was on leave. As I prepared, explained to the patient, and took consent, I was very anxious. This procedure had a potential risk to life due to internal bleeding, as the needle is bigger and we had to do it without any radiological guidance then. The doctor had to insert the needle about as thick as a ball-pen refill on the right side in the lower rib cage and then cut/suck out a tiny portion of the liver. All this while the patient has to hold his breath. Of course we used local anaesthetic, but sometimes, there may still be pain.

As I prepared the patient and started, my voice trembled while giving him instructions.

He said in his native mixed Hindi, 'Doctor, don't worry, I know you are learning. This will help you treat hundreds of patients in future. Don't worry—if something happens to me, we will never blame you. I know you are doing this for my good. If I had a son, I know he would have taken the same care as you will.'

All went well, thanks to him.

* * *

The Schizophrenic Hero

I was once posted as a resident doctor in the psychiatry ward for over ten months as a punishment for offending my HOD by praising his rival.

This bike mechanic with diagnosed schizophrenia was being interviewed in the hot Indian month of May by a smarty-pants med student, who was asking him some weird questions (students do this in the learning phase) while taking history. After a while, the student asked him, 'Do you feel there is something wrong in the way you think?' The mechanic paused and said, 'Doctor, I can say the same about your thinking if you ever repair a bike. I know there is something wrong in my brain, but that does not make you superior, does it?'

The same patient, while most other patients, doctors, and staff suffered the cruel May heat in the face of unrepaired ceiling fans, went to the dean's bungalow in the campus at 3 a.m. and demanded to see the dean, arguing with the watchman. As our courteous dean came out, the patient asked him, 'How can you sleep when so many patients in the hospital suffer this heat because of unrepaired fans?'

The next day, the fans were repaired.

A schizophrenic had done in one night what had not been done by filthy normals in years.

* * *

The Patient Who Saved the Snake That Bit Him

What to do if a snake bites you?

Well, a hundred answers, including prayers, panic, and passing out and, if possible, killing the snake. This farmer who had attended a snake-friend's lecture earlier actually decided that he would not kill the snake. He also thought (he told us later) that the snake, if at all poisonous, would have less poison after the first bite. So he followed and caught the snake (the snake must really have lost faith and confidence in its own bite thereafter!) and came with the one-foot-long green snake in a plastic bag to our ward at GMC Aurangabad.

There are various colloquial phrases in which fear can be worded, but none accurately describes the torture of sanity when someone hands you over a wriggling bag and simultaneously tells you, 'This snake bit me.'

Keeping the snake bag wrapped in another gunny bag, I gave the test dose of anti-snake venom to the patient, secured IV line and started the basic management. He was stable.

One of our dearest and most respected professors had taught us how to recognise poisonous and non-poisonous snakes. However, the medical curriculum does not teach how to handle a live snake, and they (snakes) don't understand that we doctors only want to look at their eyes, fangs, and scales closely. I kept the snake in an empty saline bottle (we had saline bottles made of glass then) and carried it home.

The patient was fine next morning. My lecturer who came for rounds gave me a weird look when I showed him the bottled live snake. He commented, 'I don't know who is wrong: you, the patient, or the snake, but there's something very abnormal about all this.' Upon asking if he could identify if the snake was poisonous or not, he pointed at the comfortable victim patient and snarled at me, *'Tyaala tari kahi jhala nahi, tumhi tyaacha chava try kara pahije tar.'* (At least the patient is safe. You try a bite yourself if you want to test it further).

You know how doctors never accept it if they don't know something!

I had equally curious friends, Dr Madhu Paulose and Dr Vijay. We took the snake to a zoology professor in the city who was also the principal of a big college. No definite answer, and we got a lot of unwanted gyan (show-off knowledge). He also drank tea alone while we were sitting in his office. We asked him if he wanted the snake for teaching. He said he could have it stuffed for the college museum. So we left with our snake friend. I was worried the snake must be hungry too.

Next, we searched for some local page-3 celebrities who were often quoted in the news as 'snake friends' and called them. All three of them gave funny reasons of why they couldn't help. So me and Vijay went out of the city and finally let out our naughty little bottled snake in the small green patch near the banks of a river. In graceful curls it ran away.

We told the patient about the snake and praised him for not killing it. His reaction was 'When it bit me, my first instinct was to kill it. Then I thought, *God has given it the bite, the fangs, and the poison for a purpose. The snake had no other option in fear.* So I didn't kill him. See, I met you all because of that snake!'

* * *

The Husband Who Turned His Wife into God

He was a diploma-holding mechanical engineer. He started his career with a big automobile-spare-parts-and-oil business. He married a girl more educated than him (arranged marriage). In three years, she developed a neurological condition that gradually disabled her completely. Regular treatment was required at bigger hospitals. They didn't have children because of this. He closed his shop, sold his house, and bought a small apartment; he started his business from within home so he could attend his wife.

He used to take her to Mumbai from Pune every three months by cab for many years. For the last five years, she had been barely able to speak or swallow. Her care and toilet had to be done in her bed. He did it all himself, starting his day at 5 a.m. and washing her, cooking, feeding, cleaning the house, etc. and also running his business. He never left her alone and arranged for help if he had to leave the house ever. I have never seen him in good clothes (he always wore the same pair), but the wife, whenever they visited us, was always dressed and groomed well. He reads on the Net about all possible treatment options, writes notes, and visits every time with a questionnaire about her condition and treatment.

Every time they visited, he carried her in his arms in my room without asking for anyone's help and not allowing ward boys to lift her because she said she didn't like it. Unlike the hyper-educated, who seek a million excuses to escape responsibilities and imbibe the 'favour' they are doing for their own moms, spouses, etc., he never made his wife feel that he is doing her a favour. He treated her as if it was his pleasure, not his duty, to attend her.

I asked him one day if he had any other relatives. He plainly said, 'I had many. They all disappeared once I became poor. Now I have only her, and for me she is God. If I have to die to make her live, I happily will. I know that there is no cure. I know that she may never improve. But I love her beyond reality.'

In these days where all men are presumed guilty because of some idiots and the term *women empowerment* has had its meaning contorted by many, there is a slim chance that anyone will notice husbands like Mr DJ who devotedly take care of their sick wives. There are a surprising many.

Mr DJ stands out among my patients.

CHAPTER 26

MEDICAL ANGELS I MET UPON EARTH: PART VI

The Mother Brain

'Get out of the ward, Rajas!' said Dr Pravina Shah.

Although many of my teachers may have thought of these very words school onwards, it was Dr P. U. Shah who finally said them in the first month of my joining the DM neurology course at KEM Hospital (Seth Gordhandas Sunderdas Medical College), Mumbai.

The issue was simple. Someone was presenting a case. I had had a terrible fight on phone with my wife that morning, so I was unable to concentrate. Dr P. U. Shah suddenly asked me about the case, and I could not answer. So she asked me to get out.

When you are a father and a postdoctoral fellow, you tend to develop a certain complex and an ego. I left the ward, angry with myself and upset with the whole world.

The next day after the OPD, she called me to the staff room.

One couldn't lie to Dr Pravina Shah. Her eyes penetrated your soul. Her brain worked superfast behind those drilling eyes, and her questions made people quiver. For it is impossible to fight a true, guileless, yet strong lady who only talks heart-to-heart. Her weapon was her fearless simplicity. You couldn't offer her anything, and she was completely impenetrable via praise. In fact, the first quality noticeable about her was a mixture of confident simplicity and a polite refusal to be pushed around by anyone. Whoever and whatever you were, you couldn't impress her except with your humble and honest good work. Her words were always kind and actions confident.

As I went to the staff room, I had wet eyes due to an anguish: that it was becoming so difficult for me to do justice to the extreme hard work required in that set-up when I was having immense stress at home, which wasn't resolving.

Dr P. U. Shah was waiting for me. 'What were you thinking about during rounds?'

'Ma'am, I had had a fight with my wife, and there were some things about my father that worried me too.'

'*Dekho* Rajas, you must first learn to switch off all the external world when you are with a patient. Whatever happens outside, let it be. When you enter the hospital, you must be 100 per cent here. Those who cannot do this will never do justice to the good doctor within themselves'.

She had told me one of the most precious things I ever learnt. To date, this has been one of the most respected commandments I practise as a doctor. There were many storms later in my life, but these words kept them outside my hospitals.

I was just another of a huge line of tough nuts she had cracked all her life. Since then, so many of her gems have made a home in the hearts of the hundreds of superb neurologists she has created over decades:

> Your troubles and responsibilities will always be more tomorrow than today. There never will be a time with less responsibility than today. So deal with today effectively—don't waste time.

> Unless you lose something, you won't win anything.

> Leave people alone. Let them do what they want. You stick to the good you have chosen.

During one of the strikes, which I was coordinating as the president of MARD (Maharashtra Association of Resident Doctors, a statewide organisation), we had planned a morcha to Azad Maidan Mumbai, and truckloads of medicos from Mumbai and all over Maharashtra were travelling there. A day prior, there were dubious phone calls with threats to my life, so some of my colleagues walked around me, covering me on all sides all the time.

Just as we boarded a truck with banners to sit above the driver's cabin, I saw Dr P. U. Shah walking towards the MARD office.

She called me down.

'Rajas, I had gone to Chembur to pray to my favourite god for your safety. Here's the prasad. Take care, and don't risk your life,' she said, handing me over the prasad and flowers. After the success of that strike, she took me to that temple to fulfil her *mannat* and donated a huge sum there in my name!

When once her husband, Mr Ushakantji, was critical in the ICU, I saw in her a wife more dedicated and caring than the ones described in most ideal books. She didn't leave his side and pulled together a thousand pieces of her sky to have one of the best cardiac surgeons do his bypass surgery. She may not like my mentioning this, but I have seen her agony and anguish in those twenty days, fighting the fate to win back her husband against all odds. For just a little help I could be to her at that time, she gifted my firstborn a gold locket shaped as her most favourite word: *aum*.

She encouraged and helped many patients with neurological disorders, especially women, to volunteer in the neurology OPD at KEM and participate in patient education. This way, it helped the patients, and those volunteering got the confidence of contributing to the society, so essential for someone with no good hopes in future.

'Stand by good. Come what may, Rajas, do good, and leave it at that,' she said often.

She also taught us to say the clinical 'I don't know' instead of beating around the medical-theory bush.

She had an extraordinary vision for her students' future. She collected the best of the people in Mumbai to teach her students. She saw to it that the external teachers were always happy with the academic environment in her department. Be it neuropsychologist Dr Urvashi Shah, neurophysiologist Dr Khushnuma Mansukhani, neuroradiologist Dr Meher Ursekar, or Dr C. D. Binnie from the world-famous Queen Square Hospital, she used her personal relations with these stalwarts to come and train us. She saw to it that we got good exposure under the genius of intensivist Dr Dilip Karnad; neurosurgeons Dr Atul Goel, Dr Paresh Doshi, Dr Trimurti Nadkarni, and Dr Datta Mujumdar; radiology chief (and probably god) Dr Ravi Ramakantan; neuropathologist Dr Asha Shenoy; and paediatric neurologists Dr K. D. Shah, Dr Surekha Rajadhyaksha, and Dr Anaita Udwadia, to name a few. She never let her personal/professional discord with anyone interfere with her students' benefits. She always encouraged us to go to other hospitals to learn and call those students to learn at KEM. In today's world where mentioning a doctor's professional rival gets the students blacklisted and environments muddy, this was an outstanding example for us.

She supervised every student's activities and attendance every day! We were supposed to call her every night at nine and inform about all cases in the ward and all referrals, get her instructions, carry them out, and only then leave the wards! Performing and reporting EEGs (electroencephalographs) and EMG-NCS (electromyography and nerve conduction studies) was almost a daily duty, and we now understand what that exposure means now!

Dr Sangita Ravat was our associate professor then (now chief). She had just returned from her epilepsy training in Australia, and made sure that we had teaching sessions every single day. Sometimes when Dr Pravina Shah was upset with a student, Dr Sangita tactfully buffered the situation. She established one of the first EEG and epilepsy surgery video set-ups in the region at KEM Mumbai and saw to it that we students were trained in it. I still remember Dr Ravat's immense efforts to get the best technology and technicians. She helped me get my overseas fellowship too.

Dr Pravina Shah regularly called all students to her home and fed them full umpteen times. Although her cook Mr Premji assisted her then, Madam was herself an excellent cook, and because I liked her *tindore ka achaar* (ivy gourd/little gourd pickle), she made it for me so many times, and I have shamelessly enjoyed it with her heavenly *theplas* while listening to her (but mostly concentrating upon the task in front of me: eating!) at her Gamdevi home balcony. She was our mother in Mumbai.

She has many proud achievements to her credit, but she never boasts about herself (another quality we learnt from her). She established one of the first epilepsy support groups in India, Samman, and again used her personal equations to get space and funds to run it. She researched with Dr Richard Masland, a father figure in the field of epilepsy. She has led the Indian Epilepsy Association and now is among its advisors too. In a world where most people boast about flying over the Everest when actually they just jump over a pebble, we never heard Madam talking about her own achievements and virtues.

We never hesitated in the face of hard work again because she made us participate in the toughest of the academic tasks. Every neurology patient admitted in ward 10 was supposed to be seen, interviewed, and completely examined by the resident doctor immediately. A forty-page pro forma had to be filled up for each patient, recording everything in the minutest detail. It was huge paperwork. The next morning, she would check each word from each pro forma and correct us. That habit has been imbibed in almost all her students.

The mud and some petty philosophies now cropping up in our profession have never affected her. She still writes the case sheet exactly like she taught us, in her beautiful handwriting. She knows the families of almost all her students and still cares for us after so many years. I have never seen her wearing ornaments, jewellery, or costly clothes or accessories. She has used most of her income to help others in various ways, never speaking about it.

In a country still struggling with the female feticide, here's the glorious story of a strong woman from a humble family who made to the top of the neurology circle in India in a field dominated by men, making not only a very successful career as an ideal doctor and teacher but also as an ideal wife at home and a mother to hundreds of students practising neurology all over the world. While doing this, she has done extraordinary social work especially in the field of epilepsy and women's issues therein. Like the tragedy of most of the honest social workers who never talk about their work, her work is yet to be recognised by our governments, which are more inclined towards sports and films when prestige awards are concerned.

But then, she does not care. Her reward is the millions of patients who continue to benefit through her students.

The loving ones who say 'Get out' to you are often the only ones who can bring you back to life.

Thank you, Dr Pravina Ushakant Shah, madam, for imbibing the strength of good upon my life, both as a doctor and as a human being!

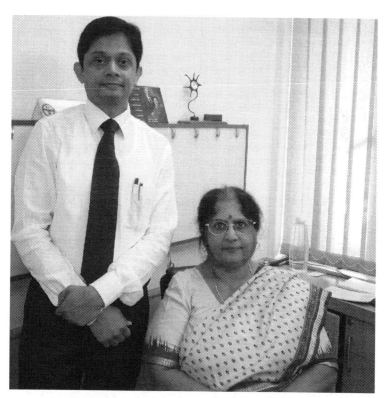

With Dr Pravina Ushakant Shah.

CHAPTER 27

MEDICAL ANGELS I MET UPON EARTH: PART VII

The Messiah of Medicine

'Sir, many times last night, I felt it was so easy to slip in some strong paralytic drug to that rapist. If that criminal is allowed to go back in the society, he will just continue to rape more women,' said the devastated intern with tears in her eyes.

We had had a tough ICU night, me and this intern, attending some critical cases along with a famous businessman who had been arrested (again) for an alleged rape and was admitted in the ICU for chest pain. He did have fluctuating high blood pressure and mild ECG changes. The intern was too affected, just like rest of the town, by his alleged crime. Our professor had come early in the morning to see him and other emergencies. While having tea after the rounds, this tearful intern said these exasperated words to him.

Dr Pradeep Yashwant Mulay answered, 'You are a doctor, not a judge. Be it a priest or a murderer, your decisions must only be for their good. You have to train yourself to keep all your judgmental attitudes and prejudices out of medical care. Even if your enemy comes to you as your patient, your only duty as a doctor is to save him and do the best for his health.'

Dr P. Y. Mulay taught us apparently simple things that were the most difficult to follow in real life medical practice, but he also showed us how to, by practising them himself. He honed the very basic medical thinking among us students.

There is a take-off point in everyone's life when they finally meet the person whom they want to be like. Everything changes there. The desire to be a good doctor can only be created by someone who dons the charisma and persona that only comes with being a genuinely good doctor. It cannot be faked. I was on the verge of quitting the MBBS course (medical school) once, wanting to pursue the spiritual. It was in the beginning of third year. Having just read the holy texts from many religions, I had lost interest in the ways of the crowds.

Then for one post-lunch lecture session Dr P. Y. Mulay walked in.

There was an actual aura of brilliance around his face! A simple, calm, soothing, but handsome personality; a smile as reassuring as a mother's hand upon one's head; the deep, heavy, and strong voice of a philosopher; and an answering style that was inimitable: a short pause after listening to the question, that sphinx-like smile, and then the perfect answer that could be to any medical or non-medical question. His eyes always contradicted the calm on his face: 'Challenge me if you can!' they irradiated.

His first lecture was about Vitamin B12. For the first time in medical years, I understood every word of a lecture without making an effort (I remember most of it even today!). Wanting to know more, I asked him few questions after the class, walking with him down the staircase. He did not show any prejudice towards me for being different in being too active in many extracurricular activities (no, I will not explain this, but all legal stuff, you know!). He was the first teacher who talked to me like I was any other student.

I started attending his lectures regularly. He once mentioned a quote from the famous novel *Final Diagnosis* by Arthur Hailey and asked the class to read it in free time. That book was not for exams, so naturally I got it on the same day and read it in a week. I had many questions again, and he took me to a nearby tea shop to answer them all. I felt alive and was mentally back in MBBS. He continued to guide me.

'You have to be like the architects of the Taj Mahal. The emperor paid for it, the labourers made it, but the conception of that idea is the most important thing about it. They imagined something so beautiful and grand that didn't yet exist. That live imagination alone can supersede the beauty of that structure that has no life,' he said when I asked him how should one plan life and career, especially with wanting to do so many things at once at all times.

I learnt this from him: What is done, achieved, is dead. The next idea in your mind is life.

'I want to do my MD medicine under him. That is my aim,' I told my scanty friends and started studying. A lower number of PG seats marred this dream for a year, and after a lot of prayers and restless nights working as a lecturer in pharmacology at Nanded Civil Hospital, I got one of the most wonderful news a doctor could get in his life: MD Medicine at GMC Aurangabad, where Dr PYM worked!

His always-happy face had become very happy because of the birth of his son Tejas by then. Wherever I was posted, I made it a point to attend his rounds, bugging him with unending doubts of a vast subject that had no syllabus! He was loved by all students, and there used to be a competition for being his favourite. He must have sensed the dire need for my resurrection, so he gave me more attention then. He had a painful spine due to ankylosing spondylitis and didn't ride a two-wheeler himself. I sensed the opportunity and selfishly grabbed it. He agreed to my request that I drop him home after the rounds, and those twenty-minute rides with him on my Bajaj super scooter were my heaven as a student; the discussions we had then have formed the basic doctor within me. Honestly, being seen around with him raised my sanity quotient among my colleagues too!

How I miss those 'Arabian evenings', where my idol bestowed upon me the benediction of medicine and of life, riding upon a two-wheeler with me! As we crossed the famous Varad Ganesh temple, I slowed down, as his home was approaching and I was never satisfied!

> Instincts are very dangerous for a doctor. Every single function as a doctor must be based upon logic and reason, and however intelligent one may be, one must never let instincts take over scientific decision-making. At least not as a student.

> There is seldom any 'classical' case of any disease: look carefully and you will find an exception to its textbook description. No two mitral stenosis cases are same. You must continuously review your findings and interpretation and make decisions individualised for every patient.

A doctor must at least know what he doesn't know and never presume. Take a second opinion, open your books, and find out your answers. If there is still no answer, be honest about it to yourself and to the patient. A doctor who thinks he knows all is a dead doctor, for medicine changes every day. There's always something more to learn about even the smallest topics in medical science.

The difference between medical confidence and overconfidence is actually life and death.

His peace was impeccable. He never lost his calm. 'You declare your mental abilities when you lose your calm. There are no problems pitted against you— there are only situations. Your emotional reaction to them, your dislike, panic, and the fear about bad outcome transform situations into problems. Stay calm, detach yourself from the fear of a bad outcome, and you will see better results.'

It is very common to see angry, shouting, arrogant, mannerless, and abusive doctors (especially successful) who take pride in showing down their own juniors, staff, and students in front of many patients/relatives, sometimes for mistakes but often to impress patients. Angry doctors upset the students, staff, and patients alike. Anger is justified only when other options of mannerful communication are exhausted. PY sir called us to the office and scolded us if we were wrong, but the scolding was always accompanied with a smile. Or he would take us to the tea shop near the hospital and explain why we must change. His love was a greater force against our committing mistakes than anyone else's fears.

He encouraged the odd and different within me, challenging me often. He gave me difficult to find topics to talk about, in that era without Internet. Once he just wrote 'MRDM' in front of my name in the seminar list. Asked what, there came that curiously naughty 'gotcha' expression on his face. He answered, 'Find out.' Malnutrition-related diabetes mellitus (MRDM) had just recently been described in India, and that seminar prepared me and my fellow PGs to deal with this difficult disease.

He taught me to infuse paclitaxel (anticancer drug) to a patient at a time that this drug was not even available in India and was imported for someone. He stood by the side of ICU patients with us to teach us the rhythm changes in cardiac patients. I remember his beautiful talks about reperfusion arrhythmias in patients of heart attack (after the clot dissolves, the resumption of blood supply to the injured area may generate abnormal rhythms in the heart, some of which may again be fatal if not treated). His recitals on Parkinson's disease, epilepsy, hepatitis, tuberculosis, etc. while we walked on holiday mornings in warm sunlight between wards are unforgettable.

PY sir saw to it that the students are never affected by disputes between two teachers. I also respect him most for one rare trait among senior doctors: he never left the side of a patient in distress or emergency. He didn't leave it to his students/PGs to deal with a critical patient. He waited till the situation resolved. His lancet-sharp presence of mind never left him. His mind was like a control centre for every situation he came across, and he was always prepared in the face of surprise.

Those days, the 'super specialty practice' had not reached Aurangabad, and we only had two. Dr Sudheer. G. Kulkarni, 'the Kidney Genius', virtually ran every day from ward to ward attending patients, performing kidney biopsies, and monitoring haemo and peritoneal dialysis patients, simultaneously teaching multitudes of students how to dialyse a patient. If Dr S. G. Kulkarni had chosen to be in private practice then, he would have defeated the richest of the rich doctors hands down, but he chose to spend most of his career doing it all free for a negligible salary, teaching hundreds of budding physicians how to deal with and protect kidneys. I am deeply indebted to him and am also in awe of this man with a mission for the kidneys of the poor, which otherwise are only cared for if they are to be transplanted!

Dr Dnyanesh V. Muley had developed himself into a cardiologist and taught us even temporary pacing of the heart in that makeshift ICU. He drove me madder then by making me prepare and study the peripheral smears and also the ECGs of each and every patient admitted in the ward. It is difficult to imagine the amount of light your past gathers and its relevance in future!

Except Dr SGK and Dr DVM, there were no super specialists, but Dr P. Y. Mulay covered for almost all of them. Although diabetes and liver diseases were his special interests, he knew so much about almost everything we asked, including our weird questions. He asked me to research about the insulin coma therapy and glucagon. He often discussed with us chapters from Sheila Sherlock's liver textbook. He was a wizard about infectious diseases, and when I was posted with him in the infectious ward, he got us a microscope to teach the hanging drop preparation for cholera bacterium along with routine bedside pathology. I remember the pride when our first neonatal (baby) tetanus patient was discharged, thanks to his perfect guidance!

Dr Mangala Borkar, one of our professors, besides being an excellent physician, was also an artist par excellence. She had made many beautiful drawings of different neural pathways and brain and spine anatomy in her ward, far before Netter's atlases were available to us. She conducted weekly CPC (clinico-pathological correlation) sessions, the most dreadful activity in our curriculum where a medical puzzle was given and the PG had to find out and justify the answer. Students were introduced to the depth of medical waters here. PY sir most usually found the answers fastest, and his academic wrestling sessions with the other professors left us spellbound, for that level of scientific proficiency was unbelievable in those pre-Internet days!

Doctors and their families spend their entire life in the shadow of deadly infections. I remember how my father broke down when I proudly told him I had volunteered to work in the plague ward during one epidemic. (Baba, of course, allowed me but was very sad for many days after that.) PY sir had always taught us: 'It is your duty to take care of yourself while treating patients. Wear mask and gloves, and take every precaution you can to avoid direct contact with body fluids, irrespective of the diagnosis. Patients are not aware if they have infectious conditions and may not tell you in some cases. Wash hands after examining every patient. Gargle with saline if someone coughs or sneezes upon your face.' These simple precautions must have saved so many of his students! There are so many doctors who suffer and some who die due to their occupation of human medical service, and I so much wish they all had teachers like him!

This son of a teacher from a humble family has gifted hundreds of the best-quality physicians to India over so many decades! I am blessed to know this 'messiah' of medicine, the mother branch of all medical specialties!

During my last year in MD, PY sir bought a four-wheeler and modified it with hand controls and seat positioning. As we once returned from a late night meeting, on the empty roads, I rode my scooter beside his van and shouted, 'Sir, is that van comfortable? You must have to drive slow with those hand controls. Does the seat hurt your back?'

He laughed. 'Let's see who reaches Nirala Bazaar first,' and he started speeding. Not believing what just happened, I raced him that 5 km chase, only to find him waiting there with a huge smile upon his face.

'All the controls are in the brain, Rajas!' he said. I realise the meaning of these words every day till date.

PY sir, please continue to bless our world with your brilliance for a thousand years more! (Okay, logically speaking, at least till you are 120 years old!) I respect, adore, envy, and love you!

PS: And yes, sir, I would like another race, please, for now I have a four-wheeler too!

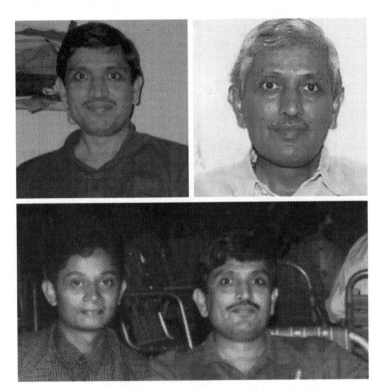

With Dr Pradeep Yashwant Mulay.

CHAPTER 28

THE MASTER

My professor's husband had a cardiac emergency and was admitted in the ICU. An emergency bypass surgery was advised, the outcome unpredictable. Madam was emotionally shattered, as they had no other family. She had always been so nice and motherly to all her students, so I decided to take leave and attend this.

Doctors are horrible patients and relatives, mostly a curse upon themselves, knowing the worst possibilities about illnesses as well as medicines (that is also why they can understand the patient's fears more than the patient).

A quick decision was to be made. Madam visited her favourite temple that morning, and we had a tense discussion. The decision was to err on the positive side; we chose the guilt of surgical risk above the guilt of fear. It is so difficult to make such a choice for someone you love!

Madam knew Dr Sudhansu Bhattacharya, one of the best cardiac surgeons in Mumbai. With a few courtesy calls, she got his appointment for that evening. We went to his clinic at the Kemps Corner. The security was unprecedented; so was the line of waiting VIPs. An entire room besides his waiting room was full of trophies, medals, and accolades for free surgeries and social causes. His secretary/receptionist was already upset with us for 'breaking in' in his tight schedule.

His room was peaceful. He was most polite and well behaved. There was a proud picture of him and his guru, Dr Dudley Johnson (one of the world pioneers of CABG/ bypass surgery), on his table. As he wrote his notes, I noticed his beautiful pen. A poor resident doctor, I was scared to ask but couldn't resist.

'Sir, which pen is that?'

'MB,' he answered, smiling, and gave it to me to try. It was buttery smooth.

'How much does that cost?' My middle-class curiosity. The other two classes do not care.

'Oh, I don't know. I guess thirty to forty thousand.' He smiled, unconcerned with that figure.

I shut up.

* * *

The surgery was scheduled next morning at Cumballa Hill. The patient was shifted there.

Madam's face reflected her torn heart next morning. I was worried about her health. One of the greatest agonies upon earth is being unable to cry; she kept up a straight face. I thought the three to four hours of surgery would devastate her outside, waiting.

'Rajas, will you accompany him inside the operation theatre?' she asked in a trembling, wet, and heavy voice. 'I will ask Dr Bhattacharya.'

I of course would! Who wouldn't want to see a master in action!

'Yes, ma'am.'

Dr Girish, assistant to Dr Bhattacharya, told us that Dr B usually did not allow anyone inside OT. He offered to put in the request for us. I waited at the hospital entrance.

The golden Merc screeched at the entrance, and the master got down. *Such a resemblance to Sir Richard Attenborough!* I thought. He walked very fast; I caught up on the stairs to him. 'Sir, can I attend this surgery?'

'Yes,' he said. 'Wash up.'

As the patient was being prepared, he asked me a few questions about resident doctors' living conditions at KEM. He softened when he learnt I stayed in the hostel. He explained the steps of the planned surgery to me like a teacher. Dr Girish joked that he was feeling jealous.

The surgery started, and the master entered the chest with the confidence of a lion. Whenever possible, he identified and showed me the crucial anatomical details. There are a few times when the surgeon has to wait for the assistant or anaesthetist to finish their part. Dr B was wearing special glasses with a headlamp. I asked him about them. He took them off and had me wear them, showing me tiny arteries that he was going to manipulate. 'You don't become a cardiac surgeon only with those glasses,' said Dr Girish, smiling. Dr B asked him to be patient with me. 'You never allowed me to touch those,' Dr G complained to him.

Dr G explained me the parts and function of the heart lung machine very courteously. He tried to keep the atmosphere tension-free in the OT.

As the heart restarted, I realised that Dr Bhattacharya suddenly became relaxed and calm. His tension was masked so well I could feel it only when it was gone. He smiled all the way through the closure.

There in that operating room, there was a doctor, an unconscious patient, the determination of a team to do good, a shadow of death, and the mystery of destiny. What came out was life, thanks to the ability of that doctor. The stress in an operation theatre can match only that of a war.

He went out and reassured my tearful professor that all had gone well.

I sipped coffee with him in the room just after the surgery. He told me about the time when he had only one pair of clothes and used to rewash them every day to wear them the next day, while staying in the hostel at KEMH and SGSMC. He told me how he had saved money by skipping meals. He told me how nobody had helped him then, adding that he had never depended upon anyone. 'I am lucky that nobody helped me then. I can make my own choices now.' He winked. No wonder he did so much charity, and no wonder no one could dictate him.

I was a nobody then, just like I am today, but he treated me like his own. That day affected me forever.

I asked for his autograph. Out came the MB.

As he scribbled me best wishes, I realised it was neither the merc nor the MB fountain pen; the real luxury was being the person that he was!

CHAPTER 29

THE DOCTOR THE DEVELOPING WORLD NEEDS MOST

'It's high time you dropped a big stone upon her head,' said the doctor.

Shocked to the core, I looked up to find all three of them heartily laughing: the doctor, the patient, and the relative.

This was a ninety-two-year-old lady from a rural area who had seen Doctor P. D. Purandare for most of her adult life as her primary care physician. She was still healthy otherwise but often complained of feeling not perfect, occasional headaches, lack of sleep, reduced appetite, etc., mostly age related-and chronic complaints resistant to most commonly used medicines. The daughter-in-law, obedient and polite but fed up with her whining mother-in-law, had asked Doctor PDP if he couldn't 'permanently cure' her symptoms. The ever-smiling, 70-year-old family physician who was known to make even patients on their deathbeds laugh, had replied, 'It's high time you dropped a stone upon her head'.

The old lady was unaffected. Education and legal awareness had not yet spoiled the friendly doctor-patient relationship by then. She touched the doctor's face with gratitude. 'I am sure I will not die as long as you are around, Doctor. Don't teach such things to my *sunbai* [*bahu*/daughter-in-law],' replied the old lady, laughing out of her edentulous mouth, a cute laughter that offends nobody, a privilege only of the very old.

I was on a vacation after my final-year MBBS exams, and having no daytime friends (explanations later), I went to one of the most favourite people in my life: Dr P. D. Purandare, a general practitioner and family physician who practised in the small and (then) backward/orthodox town of Nanded. His clinic was an open-for-all walk-in all seven days, 11 a.m. till 11 p.m. The only rule was the waiting number system. The next patient was the only VIP, whoever you happened to be.

At around every midnight, Dr PDP dropped me home after the last patient left. There was never any haste at all; the last patient got the same fresh and relaxed doctor that the first one did. Dr PDP lived his life in his medical practice. Once I asked him why he chose to practise in Nanded while his hometown was the big and developed famous city of Pune. His answer had no flavoured ego, pride, or hypocrisy: 'Because there was only one family physician here. There was a need for more, given the population,' he replied.

He had studied his medicine in Lucknow. He practised a few years in East Africa then returned to India. A scholar in many disciplines, especially music and philosophy, extremely well read, fluent in most Indian major languages, he was the only person I have seen who entered anyone's heart freely and spread joy there.

Vaccination onwards, he had grown me up to a robust health. Whenever I had holidays while in medical college, I went to attend his OPD. There was so much to learn about humanity and medicine from him. In spite of being a very scientific doctor and a royal human being, he treated everyone as his equal. I have never seen him disturbed or angry. Like James Bond, his humour sprung forth like a fountain in the most unlikely and disturbing situations, and it was only later that people realised that it was that humour that broke the ill spell on that moment. Never cheap but never also mild, his stinging comments usually made people blush. He donned the magic of good sarcasm that left no bruised egos.

He never asked for money from any patient. Most patients went themselves and paid to his assistant cum nurse compounder Hari Singh. Regularly following up patients were supposed to make entries in their own diaries about how much they owed to the doctor and pay as and when possible. People usually paid once or twice in a year; he never saw their books. Hari Singh collected the money and handed it over to Dr PDP. Of course, many people duped him. Even in that pre–cell phone era, people called him up on all days and nights and visited his home for emergency and ease both, but his calm was seldom offended.

One very poor man came with his daughter of about twenty-one and told the doctor about her constant headaches, also adding details about her financial status, that her marriage was held up thanks to his poverty. Dr PDP wrote the prescription after examining the young girl, now visibly embarrassed by her father's disclosure. The father pulled out his reluctant wallet from the depths of his clothes. 'How much?' he asked. Dr PDP, with no high-handed expression upon his face, said, 'Don't worry. You don't pay.' As the hefty farmer father started sobbing out of gratitude, Dr Purandare asked him if he could please borrow some betel nuts (supari) from him, which had accompanied the wallet from his pocket. Laughing and crying at the same time, the father gave the supari to Dr PDP and touched his feet, asked his daughter to do the same, and told her, 'This is where they say God is.'

Trust was his second nature, and patients swore by his integrity. 'It will all stay here, not with you or me,' he winked when anyone requested him to count the money. One of the best habits I learned from Dr PDP was to never count the money someone handed over in good faith.

A visibly shaking Sikh man walked in, bending forwards and walking very slowly, his actions frozen intermittently and voice almost inaudibly low. Dr PDP explained to me the classical symptoms of Parkinsonism. A decade later, learning advanced neurology in Canada, I often thought how accurate and ahead of his time was this general practitioner in a small town in India and what a sad destiny that there was no one around him then to applaud all the talent he had! This, I know even now, is the case of so many excellent clinicians, general practitioners, and family physicians in India, whose medical talent goes unnoticed and unacknowledged just because the society is yet to wake up to it.

* * *

'Your son is unlikely to survive,' I heard the physician (Dr AA) tell my parents. I heard my mother wail and my father sob, and in a few minutes, my mom was frantically calling one of our neighbours: 'Please get a rickshaw and go to Dr Purandare. Tell him I beg him to run here at once.' Mr Raghvendra

Katti, one of my father's favourite students, went in heavy rains upon his Luna moped to fetch Dr PDP.

It was just after my second-year MBBS exam. I had developed typhoid fever, and late during recovery, the fever had suddenly shot up one day and I had become delirious. My consciousness was fluctuating, and the highest antibiotics were on. Nobody could identify what was wrong. Three specialists had already asked my parents to shift me to the civil hospital ICU, fearing a bad outcome. Fever went up to 105°F.

Dr PDP came, all wet and tense. After going through all details and examining me, he asked the treating doctor to give me a shot of steroid. 'But he may worsen with steroid,' said the treating doc, who had a higher degree, and refused to give me the injection. As my mom insisted, he wrote a note on paper that Dr PDP would be responsible for any consequences. Everyone signed it. Then they gave me a shot. Within an hour, the fever started subsiding. By three hours, I was feeling better. He sat beside me, whistling.

* * *

'Chai pilao [Get me some tea].' He smiled as he told my crying parents, 'Ye saala wapas aagaya [This idiot has returned].' The physician apologised to him for the legal note. 'It's ok, Doc, he has reacted to something. Recurring typhoid fever does not shoot up this sudden,' Dr PDP said. It was later found that the IV fluid was impure. Just changing that had made a difference. (The company was later banned.)

He gave me his old Savill's textbook of clinical medicine as a birthday gift. It is one of the most beautiful clinical textbooks I ever read!

'Har Bandar ka Madaari [a street magician who handles all types of monkeys]' was his favourite expression to describe himself as a general practitioner. 'You must know the basic treatments of everything,' he taught me. Not only India but also the whole developing world needs many thousand Dr Prabhakar Dinkar Purandares today, and also the same patient-doctor relationship where the patient has equal responsibility of faith and trust as the doctor and both carry it graciously.

He initiated me during my undergraduate days into philosophy, with Jiddu Krisnamurthy, Ashtavakra Geeta, Osho Rajneesh, and then Stephen Hawking. When I told him I actually met Dr Stephen Hawking, he was as happy and proud as my father would be. He still prays, meditates, and laughs every day and makes everyone around him laugh too. He has retired and lives happily in Nanded.

Every time we meet, he turns into the master once again: 'When you realise that all the diseases and diagnoses are not in the books, you become a mature doctor. The disease in the mind is far more difficult to treat than that in the body. The young man knows the rules, but the old man knows the exceptions.' His teachings from his learned past are etched upon my brain.

Once in a very bad, low phase of life, deserted and hurt by the way I was treated by my own, I went to him and broke down. This feeling of being isolated and tortured for being different from routine is unbearable. He just sat beside me and didn't say a word till I stopped crying.

Then he said: 'Pick up the immortals among those, from whom you want approvals for being yourself.'

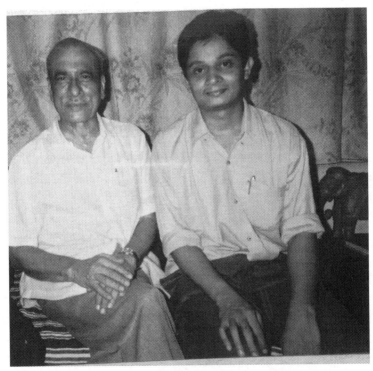

With Dr Prabhakar Dinkar Purandare.

CHAPTER 30

THE MYSTIQUE

I desperately wanted to get admission to the DM neurology course, one of the toughest known. The entrance for only six available seats in India then was attended by many hundred doctors who had passed their MD (postgraduate medicine degree). The results came on a stormy, rainy evening. There was a chance; I intensified my prayers.

The interviews left me stranded on the high edge: I was first on the waiting list for neurology. I returned with a heavy heart to Aurangabad and joined a private medical college as a lecturer, just to buy time. I started preparing for the next entrance to be held a year later. The feeling of not having what you want is the worst in the world. You know it; I don't have to explain!

A loner by nature, I sank further into studies, and my calendar was full of studying, teaching, and attending my toddler son. I was posted in a new unit. I was told the new boss would be a little 'surprising'.

I met Dr C. S. Shah, professor of medicine, next morning. He had a mocking Roger Moorish expression perpetually upon his smiling face. An excellent clinician himself, he had his own mysterious style of behaviour and speech, and the best part of it was that he was completely unconcerned about what people thought of him. Still more enviable, he didn't think at all about them.

'Why are you stressed?' he asked me one day after the rounds, as we had a light OPD. I told him I desperately wanted to get into the DM neurology course but was waiting because there were only six seats in the country then. He asked, 'So what? Study all the neurology you want and practise it . . . who is going to stop you?'

'But, sir, people look at the degree,' I replied.

'That is why you will always be stressed. People.' He laughed at me.

'Give it up,' he said.

'What?' I said dumbly.

'Your desire to do DM neurology. Give it up,' he replied with his trademark mysterious smile.

With anyone else, I would have lost my mind. But this was a person I respected.

'I won't be at peace with myself, sir,' I replied.

'Are you at peace with yourself now?' he asked innocently.

As Richard Bach says, the most simple questions are the most difficult to answer. I couldn't answer.

'Have you ever tried giving up what you desperately want just because your arrogant mind wishes it?' he asked me.

I had never. I remembered my favourite quote from Einstein's book *Ideas and Opinions*: 'Man can indeed do what he wants, but he cannot will what he wants.' Profound words by Schopenhauer!

I was not prepared to give up on this degree. This was one of my fondest wishes: to attain the highest in neurology education, and DM was an essential step for later plans.

Once we spoke about prayers, I told him my efforts and failures about meditation and Kundalini Jagruti. One of my early mentors, Dr P. D. Purandare, had encouraged me to read J. Krishnamurti, and I had attempted 'feeling one with eternity' for many times, without success.

'Because you are not prepared,' Dr C. S. Shah answered immediately. 'For feeling one with all, you cannot have a selfish intention that can harm anyone else. You eat killed animals—how will any animal feel one with you? If you take what belongs to others, if you want to be better than everyone else by showing them down, why will they feel one with you? Inner peace has a price: you cannot hurt or deceive anyone.'

It was difficult to follow this in a competitive world where the ability to cleverly deceive others is considered smartness and to diplomatically market that ability has become the gold standard for most businesses. Honesty and loyalty are considered weaknesses in a world that faces the worst addiction humanity knows yet: money.

But the divinity of good is that it seeps into your soul, whether you like it or not, and every bad ultimately learns to respect the good. I gradually started realising what a grand difference it makes to myself to not harm others by even a word, by making choices based only upon honesty and trust.

Dr Shah often told me, 'Give up your desire. It kills you. You will get whatever you want only if you pursue it with a neutral interest, with a readiness to let it go. The more you run after something, the more difficult it will get for you. Nothing is more important than your peace of mind. Don't sell it for anything else in life.'

He took me to the Ramakrishna Math (monastery), where he had found his inner peace. It was such a joy to let the silence soak your being, a flood of realisations that woke me up to what life had to offer and how my stubborn wishes had suffocated my own possible futures. To let go is not always weakness; it is also a sign of higher maturity. A loser or a coward lets go for fear, but a winner lets go for a better life.

There, in complete silence, I made a decision that a million words and thoughts had been unable to make: I wanted to move ahead, and even my best dream couldn't be an obstacle in the path for a good tomorrow.

Dreams were not meant to stop my life.

I resigned from my teaching job at Aurangabad and went to Nanded, joined one of the best hospitals there, and started working with a cardiologist who wanted to pursue a social career. He offered me to take over his hospital.

On 7 January, my birthday in 1999, I signed a contract with him. I had also finished reading the last chapter of a spiritual book on this day (Navnath Bhaktisar) as planned, and my parents were very happy about all this.

On 8 January, I received a telegram: 'You are selected for the DM neurology degree course at KEM hospital and Seth G. S. Medical College, Mumbai. Please report immediately.'

I called Dr C. S. Shah and told him I got DM just after 'giving it up'.

He laughed.

'Now give up your dream of a happy life,' he said.

CHAPTER 31

THE RADIATING PRINCIPLE

'The patient is the centre of all medical activity.'

If ever there was a *Bharat Ratna* (highest civilian honour in India) in medical sciences, the most deserving person for it would be Dr Ravi Ramakantan, ex-Chief of Radiology at KEM Hospital and SGSMC Mumbai. He created generations of excellent doctors and, besides being a genius in radiology, is also a wizard of many other medical specialties. He taught each of his students to learn from the very basic and then never stop learning.

Even after being the head, he questioned everything he himself thought and learnt, and this encouraged students to not only be humble but also keep their eyes and brains open to corrections. 'Don't treat the investigation, treat the patient,' he reminded us almost every day. He encouraged students challenging him; we never saw him offended by medical argument. He fought at times with his own friends and colleagues whenever he thought patient care was being compromised. He never accepted smart, flowery 'wise' oratory as a substitute for actual medical knowledge.

A model of simplicity, an icon of genius, and still so loving, he is respected worldwide for his crystal-clear radiology. His students practising globally are all proud of having learned from him. I was blessed recently with his visit. In an era where medical values are fading, there are people like him, even the thought of whose being clears our clouded vision.

He's a visiting professor, Brigham's and Women's Hospital, Harvard Medical School.

He was the first international visiting scholar, Radiological Society of North America, and the founding president, Indian Society of Neuroradiology.

He has received the Best Medical Teacher Award, University of Mumbai, and the Karmayogi Award, Bombay Medical Aid Foundation. He has above sixty research papers in indexed journals and over twenty orations to his credit.

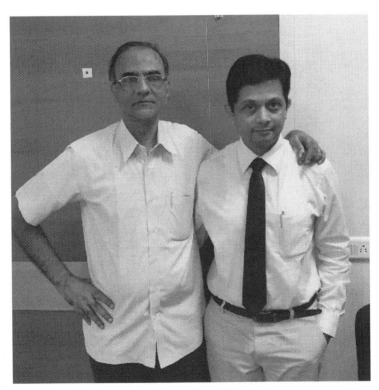

With Dr Ravi Ramakantan.

SECTION III

THE PRACTICE

CHAPTER 32

WEALTH IS HEALTH

'Please don't tell my wife, Doctor,' requested the young husband who had had convulsions and was better now, 'She does not know about my convulsions. Her sister also has convulsions, but we told nobody that our family has any such illness.'

Why? For the upper hand that he would always have over her, inducing a complex in her to get things his way.

* * *

'I am getting married, Doctor,' said this girl with a beaming smile, after the check-up.

'Great! Congratulations! I am sure you told your fiancé that you had a young stroke and are taking steroids?' I asked.

The mother interrupted, 'No, Doctor, we tried telling some because we wanted to be truthful . . . but then no one agreed to marry her. I can't afford not to marry her. She is twenty-six now and has recovered completely. Also, this prospect is very good, well settled.'

'But you will have to disclose that she has an autoimmune disease that can cause blood clots, abortions, paralysis, etc. She will face problems in the future otherwise.'

'We will handle those problems later, Doctor. Her uncle is in the police. Once she is married, I don't think her in-laws can do anything to her.'

* * *

'Doctor, my fiancé's family is coming to see you to ask about my illness. Please tell them everything is all right. Tell them that this was a one-time illness and I will not have blindness again.'

'But you may have it again. It is not something one can predict or prevent.'

'Do you plan to break a family, Doctor?' asks an angry aunt.

'No, I want to help, but a doctor must not lie or falsely reassure.'

'Okay then, we will go to our family doctor.'

* * *

'Doc, please don't tell my father that he has a cancer . . . he will be scared to death.'

* * *

'Doc, please don't write there about my real illness, but I need at least a week's leave.'

* * *

'Doc, please don't mention about my past illness, smoking, alcohol intake, drunk accident, diabetes, blood pressure, etc. in my insurance papers.'

* * *

So many illnesses that should not be hidden when fixing a match are hidden and lied about, and couples are happily married away until the 'honeymoon of trust' ends and the 'hell of allegations' reigns forever thereafter.

An illness is *not* always a patient's fault, and everyone deserves dignity, support, and best treatment. But with all this also comes the responsibility of sharing the truth that may affect any other person's life. There are rare true lovers who marry knowing completely about partner's illnesses, sometimes where one partner is completely healthy. God bless their courage and love. But there are also many cases wherein once the wife develops any major health problem, she is sent back to her parents to be taken care of, both medically and financially. I must also mention here that when the opposite happens, when the husband gets disability, mostly the wife keeps working *and* attending the husband's health issues, looking after the family and neglecting her own life, doomed to slavery.

But many psychiatric issues, neurological problems, and major childhood illnesses that can affect future health are hidden by most. Ongoing treatments are often not disclosed. Most educated people now know about common infections like HIV, HBsAg, multi-drug-Resistant tuberculosis, etc. as diseases that need attention, but beyond these there are many other health conditions that need revealing and understanding when a prospective match is being made.

Habitual lying, temper tantrums, severe panic disorder, and mood disorders form one end of this problem, while seizures /convulsions, heart rhythm disorders, liver and kidney problems, sexual/genital/skin diseases, bleeding/clotting disorders, autoimmune diseases are the other. Head injuries and surgeries in the past, abortions, and antipsychotics or some other drugs may increase the risk of future health problems in some.

While love marriages are encouraged, they are also confused with lust marriages, money marriages, and family marriages, which will never survive health storms. In a country like India, where in most cases a prospective couple does not interact with each other for more than a few 'heavily guarded by one hundred eyes' seconds, there is hardly any question of looking beyond face. No wonder, considering that there are more associations denouncing and violently attacking love rather than terrorism in our country!

There are less examples of acceptance after disclosure of a health/psychiatric issue after marriage. Mostly, divorce ensues. While the 'chill' people happily quote laws that allow divorces in such cases, nobody thinks of the scars that are being carved upon two hearts forever, scars that extend upon the face of our society! And the horror of such a marriage, if it does not end in separation but in perpetual quarrels and domestic violence, damages the future of the offspring of this unfortunate union.

The next generation suffers in many ways when health issues are bypassed in a marriage—from genetic diseases to heavy quarrels and divorce among parents affecting the kids' psyche permanently, from continuous health problems of one partner imprisoning the whole family and exploiting them directly or indirectly, to complete neglect of necessary healthcare, and so on.

No disease is bad. No patient is guilty. No doctor should lie.

In a 'health-unconscious' society, we not only need good support groups but we also desperately need premarital counselling and screening.

The society should be more open about truth, especially when health is concerned. A doctor has to respect both patients and their privacy, but if someone else's health is at risk because of a patient's health condition, the role of a doctor is not well defined. Unless sought, the doctor cannot reveal health facts—that too only with the permission of the patient. It is wise to discuss with your own doctor and accept reality.

For trust is the lifeline of any relationship based upon love.

CHAPTER 33

THE HUMANITY CULT: DOCTORS AND RELIGION

'You are in our prayers every day.' One of the greatest achievements in becoming a doctor is hearing this sentence.

But hey! You all are also there in our prayers every day!

Whatever the religion, whichever faith one may come from, whether rich or poor, whether our concepts, philosophies, or traditions match or clash, we doctors treat each patient with the same devotion: towards better health. A doctor will only ask about your religion to know your genetic risks and tendencies, lifestyle, and diet. Beyond that, no doctor thinks differently about patients from different religions. Who knows better than the doctor the oneness of the human body inside out?

We don't have to kill, sing, dance, wear T–shirts, or shout to prove our unique tradition of humanity—we carry it upon our head from the day we are born as a doctor till the day we die. Every day in every casualty anywhere in the world, the elixir of humanity flows from the doctors and nurses to the patient, and in their prayers lies the true wish of every doctor: 'Let all suffering end.'

Most of those visiting religious places ask for health and life. Doctors too work to safeguard these two, all over the world, irrespective of their beliefs. Science gives us the knowledge and experience hones our wisdom, but the prayers of millions in different religions give us the ability and responsibility to make the right choices.

Our patients, whichever religion they belong to, bring us religious gifts from their highest places of devotion. From Varanasi and Mecca; from Jerusalem and Amritsar, Ma Vaishno Devi, and Our Lady of Good Health in Velankanni; from Lord Ayyappa Temple, Khwaja Ajmer Shareef, BodhGaya, Shri Tirupati, and many other of the holiest places, I have received Lord's blessings via my patients, just like most of my colleagues I know. Abe Zamzam, the Cross, and the Holy Gangajal have blessed many of us via God's messengers to the doctor: the patients.

Any patient from any country and any religion holds some basic respect for the doctor they go to for their education and also for their presumed ability to help. This trust of a stranger is probably the greatest endangered human connection upon earth today. There is no better opportunity to serve humanity than to become a doctor. If there is any social place where everyone is really equal, it is the heart of a good doctor. There are offenders of faith and misusers of the system everywhere in the world: a few doctors and a few patients but not all.

There is so much for the doctor to learn from different religions. The art of medical practice is incomplete without basic knowledge and understanding of human behaviour, faith, and mindsets. While 'scientific' is the highest and most uncompromisable criteria for a doctor's action, this will only bring the patient health, which is incomplete without happiness. Happiness will only come from a doctor who understands human nature well. There in the wish for happiness in each mind resides the Lord. Some call it science, some God. Some do not believe in God, both doctors and patients. If themselves genuine, they still connect well via bonds of honesty, kindness, truthfulness, and mutual respect—similar foundations as that of most religions.

Many patients will not believe this, but most doctors pray for all their patients every day before starting their work. In the good of their patient lies their own good.

CHAPTER 34

WHY CAN'T THE DOCTOR BE MORE COMPASSIONATE, SPEND MORE TIME WITH THE PATIENT?

A patient-friend asked, 'When are the doctors—not all—going to grow some compassion or least show some and listen to what we actually have to say and maybe spend just a few more minutes to get to know the patient a little bit? Then maybe more patients would appreciate their doctor more. I've been fighting a disease for sixteen years now, and a lot of doctors don't even spend five minutes with you. Only speaking from many years of experience as a patient.'

Simple answer: Give the doctor a patient who writes down 'Doctor, I have complete faith and trust in you. Do your best to treat me. I promise not to sue you or blame you if in the course of my treatment something goes wrong. I respect your intention and know that you are a human being capable of mistakes. I will be compassionate to you too. I will endlessly wait in the doctor's waiting room till the earlier patient is satisfied and leaves. I am also not concerned about the other patients waiting to see you after me, and I do not care if you don't eat or sleep well.' Give the doctor a patient who pays as per time and skill required for the consult, and they will spend an entire day with that patient.

Not possible? There you are!

In the ten to fifteen years of medical training, we hear innumerable sermons about being compassionate and listening to and understanding the patient. We have always learnt and taught in medicine to listen carefully, so most doctors attempt this in practice; not all keep it up. Some learn the knack to extract the correct info to work faster.

Now imagine the doctor's side.

How long is 'a little longer'?

Seventy-five per cent of patients (including doctors when they become patients) don't have the sense of time when they talk about their illness. Instead of being to the point and realizing that this is a professional consultation, they go on to recite unnecessary overdescriptions and umpteen repetitions of the same complaints, even after the doctor jots them down. Some confuse details of their own symptoms, changing them often. Some tell their own interpretations about each of the symptoms and complete, detailed conversations that they had with their family or other doctors about those symptoms. (I had a headache, then my mom said this, then I said that, then we thought this, then my friend suggested that, etc.) Many ask the doctor to repeat long explanations twice, even thrice, then some relatives ask to repeat it again. Many revise prescription medicines at least three to four times, in spite of the doctor having written down correct instructions. Many keep blaming the doctors for the illness or poor response to medicines and crying in their cabin even after long consultations when incurable (not necessarily fatal) diagnoses are revealed, thinking that the doctor is hiding good treatment for want of more money! We sympathise and explain and want to help but cannot go on all day, especially if other patients are waiting anxiously for their turn.

Many patients fumble, forget, and come disorganised (this is super exaggerated in India, where there is no unified health record system and patients carry messed-up bundles of test reports/case sheets from many different specialists). Most (even literates) come without even the list of currently ongoing medicines then call their family from the doc's cabin to enquire about these, and then the huge discussion about spellings, content, etc. consumes double the scheduled time of consult, while other patients wait and complain. There is lack of awareness of one's own health responsibilities in many cases, and even those who spend hours chatting in the waiting room don't organise their thoughts or make notes for the consult, wasting time with the doc in recalling things!

Some talk too much; some talk very slow, take a long time to recall and answer, and mostly come unprepared for the consult without noting down questions they want to ask and symptoms/medicines they want to discuss. Then the 'recalling' time in the doctor's cabin is quite irritating for the overworked doctors. While the doctor is trained to be compassionate, their own never-ending list of tasks to finish that day makes them jittery when avoidable delays hold them. If there were a set time for every consult, more patients would be unhappy.

The third—and the most difficult—category of patients: the 'over-prepared' patients/relatives, who have hyper-googled every symptom, every medicine, and then come with a huge (and mostly irrelevant) list of questions about their minor symptoms. The stupidest of the claims on the Internet are then discussed unnecessarily, and the frightened patient/relative really tests the patience of the doctor. They are seldom satisfied with anything or anyone.

At what price?

Enter medical insurance. Enter the 'charity expectation' from healthcare providers in India, where cell phones are bought at the same price as in the USA and UK but the super specialist doctor trained in the USA/UK/Canada/Australia, etc. (with his own merit, and money) must charge as per the basic general practitioner and local sociopolitical expectations. Result: more time with each patient translates into less income worldwide.

Expectation of the society: So what if you earn less? You are a doctor. You are a spiritual saint who just earns goodwill and respect, converts that by magic into money, and then we charge you for everything, from coffee to taxes in cash! We all can dream of luxury and a good life; you can't!

A question: what's in it for the doctor in spending more (extra) time with the patient? The 'spiritual happiness' of satisfying a patient by spending more time will just add more daily hours to the already overworked doctor's day.

It is usually a pleasure for the good doctor to spend more time, explain in detail, and compassionately listen to each patient, seeing less patients and earning less for this spiritual satisfaction, but then he/she returns home to piles of unpaid bills and an unhappy family. Most medical specialists can't even afford their own home by the age of forty! Most western doctors are frustrated by the dictate of insurance companies that for a decent earning, they must see a higher number of patients. No insurance company pays a good doctor better.

As for the compassion issue, doctors feel the need to ask these questions:

1. When some doctor anywhere was prosecuted for medical negligence in some case, how many times has any patient helped him? Many doctors prosecuted must have saved hundreds of lives. Who stood by them when their careers were ruined by single mistakes? How many patients whose life they saved offered to help with the compensations the punished docs had to pay or their life thereafter?

2. How many times did society or media show compassion to the needs and plights of medical profession? Underpayment and overwork, victimisation and insecurity are universal in this profession. Who showed any compassion ever?

3. Is it possible for you to be compassionate to someone who is being a customer, with the right and threat to sue you for an amount that will ruin your life, reputation, career, and family? Can you be compassionate to someone who suspects every motive of yours, cross-checks everything you say, argues with you, threatens you, does not have faith in you, and will forget you the day their health problem is over, only to return when they need you again?

4. Can you be compassionate to someone who records your words of reassurance and uses them against you as a legal proof of 'misguiding'? Can you talk nicely to someone who treats you arrogantly and mannerlessly and looks down upon you as a moneymaker rather than a respectably educated, hard-working doctor?

Indian docs carry the whole burden of the country's mismanaged healthcare system upon their shoulders. Millions of poor, non-affording patients are, *right now*, being treated by thousands of doctors *free*. Most patients get better than not.

But when some semi or uneducated film star rubbishes the whole profession to prove themselves tall or some movie claims that doctors treat dead bodies to earn more money, no one speaks a word against it. Why?

When senior doctors who spent a lifetime serving the poor are wrongly suspended by politicians without any enquiry, there is not a peep from the society. Why?

When doctors are killed, attacked, and abused, the media justifies/glorifies such events as 'understandable reactions of angry/bereaved relatives'. Why?

Who thinks about the doctor's side of the story?

There is a worldwide notion that doctors are guilty of earning more money by wrong means like hurrying and back-door income/kickbacks. For those who think this, I have one question: which doctor in the world has more money than the price of *your* life? If they save you, they are blamed for high charges. If they don't save you, they are sued for unbelievably stupid compensations. This is the paradox: that lost lives have become costlier; saved lives don't matter any more.

There of course are a few greedy doctors who need to change. These are few and a shame. The real tragedy of our lives is this: nobody ever thinks that a doctor may really be working faster and harder to help more patients rather than to earn more money!

He/she may be struggling with his/her loans, sacrificing his/her own health and family time, fighting frustration, but still listening day in and day out to crying, angry, frustrated, complaining people merely out of their wish to relieve patient's agonies.

What price is the time you are away from your family? What price are years of sleepless nights? What price is the mental trauma of seeing dead bodies and sickness every day? What compassion did any doctor get for these from media, the judiciary, society, anyone?

PS: Less time does not mean the wrong diagnosis or approach. Mostly it means to cut off talk to bare minimum interaction necessary for this consult.

CHAPTER 35

DRUG QUALITY, PRICE, AND RISK

A doctor colleague asks, 'What about the responsibility of quality of drugs used for the treatment? These are the only weapons with which we doctors fight a disease. Does it make pharma a shareholder of responsibility in case of adverse outcome? This is another grey zone to elaborate on.'

Thank you for this question.

We must decide that we will only prescribe local cheap medicines, stents, catheters, needles, etc. approved by the government but then make it compulsory for everyone, including the ministers, government officials, actors who comment irresponsibly, etc. to only use local and the cheapest healthcare products. Let us see how many rich and famous want to use local drugs/stents/catheters for themselves or their families!

We have a society so immature that it does not blame the government for allowing production and sale of low-quality medicine and not guaranteeing and monitoring quality of each drug locally produced and marketed but thinks that the doctor should take responsibility of their 'multimillion health' by prescribing the cheapest drugs and tests available, produced locally without any knowledge of their quality!

There are set international standards of quality control for manufacturing of medicines/drugs. These apply with minor legal (but not scientific) variation to all pharmaceutical companies. Along with the major international players, there are also major/minor Indian players in this industry. Many major international pharmaceuticals have been legally tried and punished for manipulating drug-related information or bribing or compromising upon its quality—billions of dollars worth such punishments have been on record. There are no examples like this in India, which must mean the entire industry and the government's arms dealing with it must be absolutely innocent, clean, and honest, and all drugs produced in India must be absolutely good!

Secondly, the control over quality is not over with production of the drug. The transport, storage, sales, and instructions given to the patient with each single drug also matters. You know very well how many Indian drugs even have readable information printed upon them. Leave aside the separate printout labels about precautions that must accompany every sale. All this information is left for the doctor/nurse/pharmacist to educate and explain to the patient. This reduces the price of the medicine at the cost of the doctor's or nurse's time, while everyone else in this chain of sale earns their profit..

Always overworked and underpaid, shouldering many non-medical aspects of healthcare (which are the government's responsibility), the Indian doctor does not have the time, money, power, or authority to monitor, report, or check any medicines. If he does, we know what might happen. There are mighty powerful, political, medical, corporate international people who own some pharma sector, some mafia too. Can we expect a simple doctor to fight these?

I am not accusing anyone, but the two links mentioned below are enough embarrassing. We can understand that money and power can gag many in India too, from ministers to media, so these news will be rare.

<http://articles.economictimes.indiatimes.com/ . . . /47705608_1_d>

<http://www.fiercepharma.com/ . . . /indias-quality-lap . . . /2014-03-18>

There are some good and standard pharmaceuticals who tell the doctors about their quality control, ask for feedback, and also update the certifications, accreditation, etc. so we know they are standard. There are those whose brands have been internationally reviewed, those which have been in the market for decades with established safety. There are new ones with no data, where the only trust is about the maker's reputation. The onus is upon the doctor to choose. I know most doctors would prefer the best for their patients, and some would consider safety as adequate criteria if price can be reduced. Honestly, no doctor can assure the quality of a given medicine; he/she has no way to ensure that. But if you prefer local-made smartphones, perfumes, cars, etc., you may also rely upon local-made drugs, stents, or catheters. The difference is then you absolve the doctor of the responsibility of what he thinks is best for the patient.

There are umpteen examples of ineffective, low-quality tuberculosis and other drugs scandals (sold in some government hospitals) some years ago, but there was never any case decided against this.

The effective percentage of the active ingredient—its purity, its binding with the excipients, its bioavailability after consumption, its effects on the liver, kidney, brain, eyes, heart, etc. are all also linked to how much and how rapidly it is absorbed and metabolised. The doses we use are all Western-standardised, and we have a tendency (even in medicine) to presume that Western biostats will exactly apply to all population, irrespective of genetic, ethnic, and cultural differences.

A drug may kill (either by its action or inaction) if its quality is not accurate, and this quality *no* doctor knows.

It is easy for film stars who shoot outside India, drive foreign cars, endorse foreign brands, wear foreign clothes, and run to foreign countries for every health issue to cry on national TV and urge everyone to use generic local drugs. It's not their life, and if something happens, there's always the Indian doctor to blame!

The simple law 'Do unto others as you would have them do unto you' is conveniently forgotten by some who advise what they cannot themselves follow!

CHAPTER 36

DO WE HAVE A PARENTING IQ?

Parenting is the most difficult career. I don't know when it became unfashionable for some who claim success 'outside' parenting.

However successful one may have been otherwise, if they have neglected growing kids for want of money, fame, or career they have committed a crime.

There is no greater insult to childhood than a parent *not* having time to spend with kids. The only exceptions may be military services or selfless (not for any personal gain) sacrifice in the larger interest of humanity.

Equally guilty are the parents who carry home the fatigue, stress and irritation related to their work and claim that the family has to bear it as they are earning or expect the non-working parent to cover for both.

Childhood is a magical, most enjoyable phase in life, and any parent who has sacrificed his/her career for raising children is more respectable (even if less literate) to me than the ones who sacrifice parenting duties for a better material life.

Providing for family's needs is essential, but the greedy option of earning more to give them best (which is never enough) and in the process killing the option of spending time with the kids is so unintelligent!

One should consider and discuss with their proposed match before marriage about their individual 'parenting IQ' and the distribution of career choices/duties so that one parent at most times—and both at many times—are available to attend the children.

Only the mother or only the father are *not* the options; neither are guilt-ridden, compensatory annual family vacations.

Children are happiest when both parents are with them together; it is so sad that the grown-ups rarely understand this. Most working parents would argue that this is so impractical. Hence the title of this article.

CHAPTER 37

THE UNSAFE PILOT/ DRIVER: WE DON'T EVEN GRASP THE THREAT!

Imagine someone without self-control handling a gun around you or driving a truck/train or flying an airplane with you in it.

The recent claim about a pilot 'deliberately' downing his plane with many others will make most neurologists/psychiatrists recall the horror every time they advise a patient not to drive and the patient flatly refuses, quoting reasons like his/her income is dependent upon driving, it is only a short distance, etc. or just smile away diplomatically, meaning 'I don't care, I will still drive.' There was a recent tragedy in an Indian metropolis where a bus driver went on a spree that killed many.

Is it possible that the pilot was conscious and could move but was not in control of his/her actions? Yes, there are some types of epilepsy where this may happen (e.g. complex partial seizures). There is a condition in a slightly elder age group, called transient global amnesia, where the patient is fully conscious, behaves apparently normally, but has no memory of an entire time period lasting few minutes to hours, during which they may drive, perform routine tasks, etc. It is debatable whether a correct and determined sequence of actions is possible during such seizures or TGA, but this is not unknown. Also, some drugs may cause abnormal behaviour, pushing the patient over their edge of normalcy. While depression may cause harm to self or others, it is rare for that - level of depression to suddenly emerge or be unnoticed. There are usually clues in speech and behaviour about such intentions weeks prior to such action.

There are some medical conditions incompatible with driving, flying, adventure sports, swimming, and in general, being in charge of public safety. These include epilepsy, any episodes of recurrent unconsciousness due to any cause, having had large strokes in brain, having had open-brain surgeries, heart diseases with abnormal rhythms or clots that can precipitate unconsciousness, uncontrolled blood pressure (that can lead to bleeding in the brain), medicines that can cause abnormal behaviour or can precipitate convulsions and psychiatric derangements etc. Some infections in the brain may also cause sudden abnormal or violent behaviour. Most of the medicines used for treatment of epilepsy, anxiety, psychiatric conditions, allergies, muscle relaxation, etc. are notorious in causing drowsiness. Many of these conditions are beyond recognition of even general practitioners or specialists untrained in these diseases. There are hundreds of people out there with poor physical self-control (like balance disorders, Parkinson's disease, stiffness or weakness in hands or legs, impaired vision, daytime somnolence, etc. Imagine the threat to kids, pedestrians, and other vehicles with even a slight delay in braking!

While some educated/socially responsible patients agree and stop driving, many just laugh away the instruction. Besides alcohol consumption and withdrawal, some other factors also increase the chances of unconsciousness/convulsions, like lack of sleep (most truckers drive at night, at least in India), fasting, severe stress, fever, and some over-the-counter medicines like cough syrups, etc.

One can understand and sympathise with the need of the poverty-struck class to have to work for survival, but the risk this causes to general public is unacceptable. Hundreds of accidents kill thousands of people on the roads every day, and it is high time we think about this.

What can be done?

In most countries, including India, patients with seizures are permanently banned from driving and piloting. In some countries, a certain seizure-free period is compulsory before the license can be reinstated. However, in India, this is not at all implemented, as the doctors are not authorised to retain the driving license of the patient at the first hint of risk. This is a standard procedure in all developed world, and this is usually done with caution as many patients protest and some get violent too. It is very difficult, given the Indian society, which not uncommonly beats up even the traffic police for stopping them and calls politicos, senior police officials, and judicial staff to suspend or transfer anyone who interferes with their free, drunken driving. However, the doctors must have forms and hotline numbers where they can at least report potentially dangerous drivers.

It will be interesting to know how many driving licenses were rejected in India quoting seizure disorder, alcoholism, psychiatric conditions, or other medical reasons: the prevalence of seizures is one in every one thousand population!

Most airlines take a normal EEG (electroencephalogram, which records electrical activity of the brain) test as an evidence against epilepsy. However, this is an elementary test, and a normal EEG does not rule out epilepsy. Only qualified neurologists, epileptologists, or psychiatrists can identify some types of seizures.

While it is impractical for a driving or flying license applicant to visit many specialists, the criteria of basic medical evaluation can be definitely upgraded, and the screening doctors can be trained better in identification of potential risks.

The educated and socially responsible should voluntarily refrain from driving if they have these conditions and resume only when their doctor allows them.

Let us spread the word for our own good.

CHAPTER 38

THE SECRET INGREDIENTS OF A HEALING TOUCH

Most doctors in the world are good. Some are extraordinarily good, some below average.

Here are some factors that I think make an extraordinarily good doctor. As far as possible, I have tried to mention them in the order of their importance, but the sequence is not much important.

Extreme compassion for all humans and other life forms is almost mandatory. Suffering of any patient must be understood and resolved in the best possible manner, irrespective of all their other qualities, however much the doctor may dislike them as a person. Once you put on the white coat, there is no bad patient. To relate a beautiful observation, most doctors in the world, even when chronically underpaid, do not differ in their treatment plans whether the patient pays or not. Added compassion makes it sweeter.

The number of patient-years matters: more the number of patients treated, wiser the doctor becomes in that given specialty, up to a certain age.

A commitment to continue to study is crucial. Every day, each doctor comes across at least one question in his own analysis or posed by a patient or student that they cannot answer. New medicines are added every day, and the higher you grow in your field, the farther away remain the advances in other fields. One to two hours of self-study like a graduate student every day is typical of an excellent doctor.

One must try and concentrate upon understanding each and every thing relevant about a patient: complaints, examination, test results, ongoing medicines, and the interplay of these factors. All possible question marks should be erased from one's mind as soon as possible. Fortunately, the Internet is a boon here. 'To treat in a hurry' is the trademark of lurking danger ahead.

There is a tendency to accept mistakes, rethink, and review one's own conclusions, to discuss them with colleagues time and again. This is especially important if the patient does not get expected relief with a given line of treatment. A doctor who thinks he/she is always right and knows everything is not only wrong but dangerous.

In the days of rampant medicolegal blackmails, it is difficult for the doctor to be too honest in discussing things clearly with the patient/relatives for fear of being sued for even minor mistakes, thanks to the legal twists. Still, one must at least try and use acceptance of mistakes for doing good to the patient.

There must be a confident stance to stick by the truth, even if one cannot explain it fully. The basis of all medical thinking must be scientific reasoning alone. In a world that has cleverly evolved to misuse logic and reasoning, this is becoming more and more difficult. 'Evidence-based' is not always universally applicable to all. A certain depth of clinical analysis, interpretation, and application is essential; otherwise, the doctor tends to become a *Pubmed Peter*, quoting umpteen references for everything but unable to satisfy the patient.

A strict discipline of body and mind is essential. Doctors live a very rewarding life but are exposed to much more physical and mental abuse by an over-expecting society, which is reluctant to understand or solve their concerns. Add to this daily exposure to death, suffering, illness, panic, shock, allegations, laws, competition, and the stress of always having to make correct decisions. One must learn to 'switch off' the external world when with patients. This is difficult when you yourself or your family members are sick or if there are other issues that disturb you. It is wise to 'call it a day' and not work (unless an emergency) if you are not feeling well. Adequate rest, sleep, food, and exercise to maintain yourself in good health reflects as your commitment to offer the same to others.

The second part of this discipline is the concentration with which one must grasp every word that the patient or relative says, to pick up every possible abnormality upon mental and physical examination and various tests, and to analyse and reanalyse it all in one's mind in the most logical manner to come to a conclusion, diagnosis, and its closest other possibilities (differential diagnosis). If an intervention/procedure/surgery is planned, a complete individualised profile of the patient must be imprinted upon your mind, with your plans and contingencies, post-operative management, and follow-ups. As one grows up, one's capacity multiplies in remembering these details.

Giving every patient detailed instructions about diet, exercise, sex, physiotherapy, lifestyle, addictions, medicines, sleep, and travel during discharge is a mark of a truly complete clinician. Swiftness, speed of accurate decision-making, and presence of mind (mindfulness) is uncompromisable for a good doctor.

A very positive, hopeful mindset, always giving the patient the extremely important feeling of you 'being concerned and hopeful' about their good health outcome, is necessary. The medicolegal mess prevalent today is killing this concept, but a wise doctor should learn to explain the 'risk' part in a compassionate rather than amplified manner. A kind, non-committal reassurance and addressing the fears in direct words goes a long way.

Respect for patients and their decisions to not take treatment, to disagree with you, and to obtain a second, third, and umpteenth opinion cannot be questioned. You may refuse to see that patient again and charge higher for more time or review, but your behaviour should always show utmost respect for the patient. Understand that almost every patient is frightened within and seeks reassurance but is too proud to ask for what is essential. A patient afraid to face his own fears reacts angrily and behaves irrationally, and often, the doctor becomes the target for such patient's anger. One must take this in his stride and still be able to retain a kind and understanding attitude towards the patient.

A determined control over negative emotions, especially anger and grief, is difficult but essential. These two are constant companions of a doctor. Bereavement caused by one's patient's death causes immense mental trauma to many doctors. Allegations, stress, arrogance, and angry relatives are commonplace. Amidst all this mess, the doctor must also deal with a normal worried patient every day, who expects the doctor to be smiling, fresh, attentive, and receptive then reassuring.

A regular short vacation is very essential for a doctor chronically exposed to such heavy stress. This kind of stress is worst among surgeons, interventionists, paediatricians, intensivists, neurologists, and oncologists, but every doctor is either a minor or major victim of severe stress.

The appearance and bearing of their doctor are very important for the patient. One must always be dressed up professionally, practise the local traditions, and behave with the best manners, preferably with international etiquette. An apron may make some paediatric patients anxious, but in most cases, it reduces the 'stranger' feeling about the doctor. A clean, healthy, well-groomed, well-behaved, and smiling doctor with an aura of freshness definitely encourages the patient's confidence. Clear, calm, honest, non-hurried, and confident speech matters a lot when counselling the patient. Negative words, defaming colleagues, vulgarity, cheap talk, gossip, too much money talk, joking about the patient, neglecting the patient, and anger are all turn-offs for a patient's faith in their doctor.

Effective communication goes a long way too. In properly chosen words, one must explain to the patient everything that they want to know about their illness, in sessions if necessary. Educating and encouraging one to learn about one's illness assures compliance and reduces misunderstandings.

Being there for all concerns is important, albeit with appointments and proper channels. Patients who develop faith or liking for a doctor often confide in them about their spouse, family, etc. and expect help to untangle personal life. Solving what one can and referring the patient to the right specialist if one cannot help falls well within the Good Samaritan duties of a doctor. Sometimes a patient may develop feelings for his/her doctor, or vice versa, this is best addressed outside the medical practice. Just because they are in a hospital, they do not cease to be human. Such issues need extremely delicate approach, and the rules in some Western countries are a good guide for such a situation.

Being a good teacher, encouraging juniors and students to learn, and teaching them by example form the basis of the excellent traditions of medical education. Technology will never replace clinical discussions and analysis. Medical students, like most others, are too wise to be preached what the teachers themselves do not practice.

Money and affluence is as essential and necessary for a doctor as for anyone else. A doctor must strive for a good and productive life without feeling guilty for a desire of affluence. However, while earning what one wants, one must never compromise on the quality of their work. As a community, doctors are better evolved among the educated and should not await for a 'slower' social mindset to catch up with a doctor's needs and plight. Money should neither be a guilt factor nor a decision-making factor about a patient in a doctor's life. The means of earning it had better be honest, and patient's trust is the most precious commodity we earn.

There are many more, like spirituality, the knowledge of dealing with death and the bereaved, the knowledge of the good and bad research, the wisdom that comes only after being exposed to multiple complex situations, a graceful acceptance of helplessness in the face of irremediable adverse situation, and an impetus to understand human nature, to stand kinder and taller than oneself, that all go into the making of this rare creature: a doctor with a healing touch.

The only element of magic in any doctor's healing-touch potion is the blood and sweat shed in their extreme hard work for many years. The sacrifices that a doctor makes can unfortunately only be understood by another doctor!

CHAPTER 39

THE POISONOUS MEDICOLEGAL BREW

'Doctor, we think that doctor treating my mom is giving her the wrong treatment. She has been in the ICU, unconscious, for the last three days,' said the angry and crying son.

A nice fifty-five-year-old lady farmer with epilepsy, well controlled with two medicines, without fits for last three years, had suddenly developed many fits/convulsions at home, and was now in the ICU, ventilated because of the necessity to paralyse to control fits (a common recommended treatment). Her brain had suffered damage due to lack of oxygen, as breathing was compromised during fits.

As per their request, I called to talk to the doctor treating her. She courteously explained that the patient had been admitted after many convulsions, in an unconscious state, and with dangerously low oxygen levels. The management since admission that she narrated was the correct one recommended in this case. 'We will try to wean the patient off the ventilator tomorrow,' she said.

Ten days later, the patient visited my OPD with her sons. Having known me earlier, the emotional lady held my hands and cried a while, thanking God for her rebirth.

'What happened on that day?' I asked her.

'Oh, I missed my antiepileptic [fits] medicine for five days,' she said.

'Why?' I asked, agitated. We clearly explain to every patient the importance of taking medicine regularly, on time, and about stocking extra too.

'I live in a village. My son sends me this medicine from Pune. This time I told him a month earlier, but he couldn't send it as he was busy,' said the ever-forgiving Mom.

I looked at the son. He said, semi guilty, 'Doctor, I thought four to five days of break in treatment would not make a difference. Also, some people tell us that sometimes doctors prescribe unnecessary medicines for years, so we were confused whether she should continue. She had not had a convulsion for three years too.'

'Then why did you blame that ICU doctor when you saw me last?' I asked, still sizzling inside with hurtful anger.

'You can understand, sir, we were emotionally disturbed as Mom was critical. Also, we had to spend a lot for her treatment.'

* * *

A case of brain cancer, stage 4.

Her headache had been neglected for three years. A doctor had advised MRI, but that was delayed, too, for months. Then it was done when she fainted. Multiple brain secondaries had caused a block to the flow of brain water (CSF). She was operated in emergency by one of the best-reputed senior neurosurgeons to restore the life-saving flow of CSF and obtain biopsy. It proved to be a stage 4 cancer. Radiotherapy was started, but the patient ultimately succumbed. The relatives kept on asking, 'Was the neurosurgeon wrong? Was the surgery done correctly?'

Where do we bring faith and trust from, in this world where even brothers, sisters, and parents are killed for money and most couples find it difficult to respectfully trust each other?

Some patients often expect a miracle from someone they don't trust.

In the widening valley between patient and the doctor, where trust is paramount, some media and television shows have further created a rift that has inflicted severe damage. This poisonous medicolegal brew has really caused immense corrosive effect on this beautiful profession of intellectuals. Like other cheap 'filmy' philosophies, this whole allegation game neglects the very high standards of education, compassion, and sacrifice practised by 90 per cent of the doctors worldwide.

Of course, a logical analysis is not to be expected from someone not well educated. Many celebrities have been victims of the 'genius grandiosity' that money and fame brings.

The effect of this poisonous medicolegal brew:

Many—if not most—patients now enter the hospitals with suspicion in their mind and aversion for the entire process of consultation, paying fees, investigating, admission, and taking treatment, all of which is a natural, healthy process followed worldwide in all hospitals. Indian patients are unaware of how good the available specialist medical services are, at least in the urban/semi-urban areas, at the lowest costs anywhere in the world. Just because there are a few unfair practices and greedy doctors, so many others suffer, doctors and patients too!

It takes up to two years to get an appointment of specialty surgeon—over a year for a neurologist, one year for a cardiologist, three months to do an MRI in some parts of the developed world. These can be expedited only in an emergency, where one cannot have the choice of a specialist. This is mainly because they work 8 AM to 5 PM OPDs. Even senior docs in India work late nights and earn one-tenth or less, in most cases, to be available for anyone within a day, irrespective of their financial/social status.

The notion that everything best in medical care should also be free is damaging the future of this profession, especially in India. Add to this the loose talk by some celebrities and other socially influential intellectuals who have great hold on the illiterates/semi-literates. People who are already angry at the government, at their own poverty, unemployment, etc., find the intellectual, hard-working, and comparatively better class of harmless doctors an easy target to screw for their personal frustrations.

The poisonous medicolegal brew is not a surprise, for it definitely stems from frustration due to unexpected illness, expenses, and death. What surprises is the willingness with which both the illiterates and literates swallow it, not knowing how harmful it is for themselves.

CHAPTER 40

THE GUARANTEE OF LIFE

'What is the guarantee, Doctor?'

The best of the doctors internally react like metal on sandpaper to this apparently innocent question by the patient or relatives. While surgeons are the most common victims of this question, physicians also often succumb to these words. It's not that the doctor wants to hide or lie; it's just that the real answer is too complicated to explain to everyone in these days of word-by-word legal scrutiny and over-interpretation of colloquial reassurances. This question was earlier asked only in context of surgical outcome but now is asked with reference to outpatient treatment, hospital admissions, and any planned or emergency treatment.

A simple example—a patient developing a heart attack in the OPD is advised to get admitted and start treatment in the casualty. Patient is very anxious; so is his family.

The panicked wife asks, with tears flowing, in front of the patient, 'Is it very serious, Doctor? Will he be OK?'

'Yes, please go to the casualty immediately,' the doctor says, meaning to reassure.

'Guaranteed he will be OK *na*, Doctor?' asks the patient's son.

'I cannot guarantee, but we need to start treatment immediately.' The doctor is on guard now.

'What are the percentage chances of his recovery, Doc?' asks the suspicious son.

What should the doctor answer? A few years ago, a confident and reassuring 'Don't worry, he will be all right, just admit him and start treatment quickly' would have been sufficient. But today, one can't use these words in presence of a family recording one's conversation or having no prior exposure to the basics in healthcare and heart attacks, as 'The doctor said he will be all right and misguided us' is the hanging legal sword. Also, the truth that 'the patient is having a heart attack and is in a potentially critical state' told with any amount of compassion, concern, and love is going to worsen the patient's anxiety and blood pressure and thereby risk his health further.

If one tells the truth about possible complications of a heart attack, including death, there are also the allegations of 'overinflating the risk to get the patient admitted and get the investigations and earn from this-and-that treatment, angioplasty, or bypass surgery, which may be unnecessary'!

Most diseases have standard manuals and treatment protocols, which most doctors follow. But if everything medical was this mechanical, patients could choose their own medicines by researching through Google and also hire robotic machines to get their own surgeries done (and I am sure robots will not mind being beaten up or sued for failure). When one expects human skills, one must also accept human limitations and mistakes.

The best team of doctors anywhere in the world will never be able to guarantee the life of any human being for any period of time. With all investigations and check-ups, the best guarantee one can receive is 'At the present moment, you do not have any apparent condition that threatens your life or health, and with a reasonable confidence, we think that you should be able to tolerate x amount of stress for y type of procedure.

We cannot exclude the possibility of your developing any reactions or complications to a procedure/single medicine or a combination of more medicines.'

Many patients are understandably afraid of admission and surgery. Most physicians/surgeons are equally concerned about the outcomes. Mostly, the patient chooses a doctor whom he can trust. So where does it all go wrong with the *guarantee* word?

No one can explain everything that happens in the human body or even why and when exactly things go wrong in some diseases or in a particular case. Most of our current medical knowledge is based upon centuries of research, but what we don't know far exceeds what we know. In spite of the best drugs used, the patient's body may not respond the same way in all cases. Patients may develop fatal reactions to the simplest of the common medicines used in the OPD or hospitals. ('Wrong Medicine Given by Doctor Claims Life', says the media.)

Medical literature quotes many instances of sudden cardiac arrest (stopping of heart), sudden severe drops in blood pressure, respiratory arrest, convulsions, etc. during even the simplest of the surgeries/procedures like dental surgeries. Although every procedure with risk must be planned in a set-up prepared for resuscitation, no one can guarantee a good outcome of resuscitation. Apparently healthy, improving patients may develop sudden complications, and then the suspicion and blame game begins.

Given this, any doctor who predicts a guaranteed good outcome or percentage of recovery is actually stating the statistical possibilities based upon her experience for that specific patient and that specific treatment or procedure. These are never hard-and-fast assurances of definite outcomes. Consent letters signed by the patients or relatives mention most of the risks involved with procedures/surgeries, including death.

However, for the non-surgical cases, there are no consent forms for treatments and accepting the risks of their failure/adverse effects. Therein results the over-expectation that any non-surgical case, especially in the young, must only get better.

While every doctor must explain all possible risks, minor and major, and encourage the patient to read standard websites about the risks and outcome statistics of the planned procedures, this is highly impractical in a country like India with the majority illiterate and superstitious population. The mention of true risk/death risk, however minor, may end up in the patient deciding against surgery or medical treatment. Not every patient or relative is a stable-minded, intelligent philosopher who can analyse and accept the situation, and a negative reaction about the doctor telling them the truth is quite a common scenario.

'In this advanced age, why can you not guarantee a good outcome of a surgery and so many diseases, Doctor?' ask some innocent worshipers of *Discovery* and science channels and Holly Medical TV serials.

Hmm. Spaceships fall or fail even today. The US president's and security agencies' web accounts are hacked. Hundreds of earthquakes happen without any prediction in spite of thousands of satellites. The richest of the people treated in the best of the hospitals in the world still die. Hundreds of rapes and murders happen every day. Traffic accidents kill thousands daily. Pilots still crash their planes in mountains with hundreds aboard. Does advanced technology prevent all these? Does anyone guarantee a definite punishment of a murderer or rapist who committed the crime with multiple witnesses? Can we guarantee proper electricity, rain, weather, and food for all with all the advances in technology we have?

Why quote these examples?

Just to show that unless the risk directly affects one's self or family, the limitations of technological advances are comfortably accepted.

No one has become a better human being with any modern technology.

Like everything else controlled by nature, the human body is mostly unpredictable. Mood, sleep, behaviour, and digestion are all unpredictable even without external influence. Add one external factor—say, stale food—and all the above change unpredictably. What is so dangerous about this uncertainty?

Although these examples below are rare in the general population, they are quite common in the medical establishments:

Otherwise healthy people of any age may have a tendency for abnormal rhythms developing in the heart. They may already have 'stenosed' or constricted blood vessels in the heart or brain, which may shut down during procedures because of high or low blood pressures. They may develop blood clots spontaneously or in response to infection, immobility, or dehydration. The heart may stop suddenly in response to some commonly used medicines; it may also dilate and fail to pump in severe stress. There may be ballooning of blood vessels in the brain (aneurysms), which may rupture either without apparent cause or with even minor stress or high blood pressure. There may be a tendency for convulsions (even when the patient never had them in earlier life). Even with regular medicines like antibiotics, anaesthetic drugs, and contrast media used in some CT scans, etc., patients may suddenly develop a flurry of seizures. Hospital admission and surgery are both stressful states for the mind, and patients may develop higher blood pressures in the hospital or around the surgical day.

Some people may have kidney/liver/nerve/spine/brain damage just on the verge of failure; some may have increased chances of developing an infection due to low immunity, and the chances of catching dangerous infections in the hospital environment are always higher. Before any minor/major surgery, the doctors' team usually thoroughly does the standard check-ups required to minimise risk for that procedure; the budget given to the patient includes these tests too.

To express in simple terms for the highly-software-savvy younger generations, if at all we make a software for eliminating all risks and do all the tests to ensure good health and outcome prior to surgery or for the treatment of any medical condition, even then, the risk will never be shown as zero, although the cost of completing this for even a minor surgery would exceed five lakhs and take two weeks minimum. Also, the software will automatically increase the risks with delay in starting the treatment, smoking and alcoholism, diabetes and hypertension, genetic factors, and many other factors. It would be far more than the 10–30 per cent risk to life that the skilled doctors usually predict during major surgeries and would also reduce the 80–90 per cent guarantee they assure for a good outcome of many major surgeries.

Without such software, the doctor's brains, experience, and skills will have to be trusted for risk assessment and prediction based upon their training. These, to state honestly, are not always the best when cheapest.

To state bluntly and begging forgiveness, the current informal deal is 'Doctor, do the best you can in minimum expenditure with a guarantee of life and good outcome.'

One cannot even guarantee if one will reach home today, what with traffic and terror. We accept that anyone can die any time due to a natural disaster. Similarly, our society must also be educated that just reaching the hospital is not a guarantee of life or cure. While most doctors take utmost care for a good outcome, things may still go wrong, more frequently in a hospital.

There is no justification of negligence. Every mishap must be questioned, investigated, and explained, but the presumption that all mishaps in a hospital are the doctor's fault has to go. The investigation of any such complication must also include health information hidden by the relatives or patient, delays in investigations and treatment advised by doctors earlier, addictions and adherence to prescribed medicines, interference in treatment by seeking multiple opinions, treatments from various pathies simultaneously, and involving non-specialist doctors. It must also involve the delays by insurance companies in sanctioning the funds for which relatives keep on postponing the tests and even treatment.

If truth is palatable, legally speaking, there are no guarantees in medicine. Only good and bad chances may be predicted by experienced doctors in that specialty, that too approximately. As long as legal fears interfere with medical treatments, patients will continue to suffer.

By the way, what do we guarantee to a good doctor?

Ask the thousands of burnt souls practising medicine only for its spiritual rewards.

CHAPTER 41

CURE THIS HEADACHE

This young woman in her early thirties complained of severe headaches. She was accompanied by a caring but frustrated husband and two sweet kids. One was withdrawn and cranky while the other one was hyperactive.

'These headaches started only after shifting to this city five years ago,' she said. They were from a state far away.

'I am usually fine on holidays, but on almost all other days, I wake up feeling sick and without energy, and even a small factor like bright light, loud noise, or reading brings on the headache. It then becomes so severe that I have to sleep or take painkillers. I can't sleep every day, so I take this painkiller daily. Even a little stress at work makes me very irritable, and when I return home, I have no energy left to do anything. We have started fighting a lot,' she said, looking at her husband with wet eyes. 'I know he is tired of my headaches, but what can I do? We have seen so many doctors in so many places.'

'She used to be very happy when we married, Doc,' said the husband. 'I feel this is a totally different girl now. I do everything I can to help her, but I have work pressure too.'

Nuclear family. Both working six to seven days. Both on highly responsible posts. Long hours. Changing shifts too. Kids attended by maids when not in a day care. Their parents on both sides far away. They have had two kids with a very short interval between them, so their 'growing up' was almost together.

'Is it possible that one of you changes their job?' I asked this very cautiously, almost knowing the answer.

'No, Doc, our current jobs have excellent prospects and incomes too,' said the husband.

'Can you change the timings so you get an hour's rest without having to attend any tasks?'

'I can't change the timing. I don't think I am stressed. My husband helps me a lot by cooking and looking after the kids. It's a daily affair now. If these headaches are gone, I will be all right.'

The caring husband, who was until now attending both the kids, especially the hyperactive one, said, 'I have suggested her that she can take a break, but she wants to continue as she thinks she will get bored at home.' He threatened the hyperactive one, now climbing upon my table, with his hand.

I explained that the habit of taking painkillers may itself be worsening the headaches, in addition to the dual stress at work and home. All said and done, a woman usually attended two jobs when she worked. I also enquired if they could have their parents stay with them alternately so things will be better arranged at home.

'They don't get along well with us, Doc. My parents irk him, and I don't get along well with his parents too. We have had a love marriage. Sometimes I feel like ending my life.' She started crying.

Her examination was completely normal.

As I wrote the notes, I wondered how many of these things were correctable. Nobody wanted *gyan*/philosophy or counselling. No amount of medicines was going to take away the basic problem: a lifestyle without rest or peace and no time for love. What happens to a relationship where there is no more gelling of the husband and wife, of parents and kids, because they don't get time to be together?

One of my yoga teachers, Mr Mohandas (at the Kaivalyadham Centre on Marine Drive Mumbai), always told me, 'When you mix the sample curd and milk, it will not all become curd immediately. It has to stand for some time before the mixture forms new curd. Any relationship that has to mature into something meaningful will require quality time spent together, both with and without the kids. This time has to be separate from merely eating or sleeping together or travelling for work. Fast friends who fall in love and marry end up in tangled fights after becoming too busy, sucked up in the work and family routine so much that they become strangers again.'

Everything for a good life was at their footstep, but life itself had taken a vacation for lack of time. Bodies change, and so do minds. Too much company becomes an irritating nag. The need for personal space is disputed if at all recognised. Meditation is not truly possible when chores keep knocking at the door.

As I advised her some medicines and yoga, I could not help but suggest her that they both needed to rearrange priorities in life.

It was not my place and these are not the times that one can 'politically correctly' suggest the right priority options, but kids growing up neglected because both parents are either working or tired is certainly not a healthy option. Lifestyle choices should not take childhood for granted.

We desperately need this law: that at least one parent must spend a few dedicated hours with his kids every day, quality time, without being exhausted or irritable.

I wished the mother well via my prescription, but my heart was with those two kids.

For what those two kids were unknowingly suffering is beyond our society's conscience to deal with, and beyond its maturity to logically talk about.

CHAPTER 42

THE LAWLESS SIDE OF MEDICINE

A fifty-some-year-old, a well-educated and powerful businessman driving in his car with his family, had an accident. His hand and forehead had some bleeding wounds, but he was fully conscious and alert after the accident. A few young college-going students stopped to help, picked him up, hailed an autorickshaw, and took him to the hospital. The patient's wife and child followed in another autorickshaw. The junior surgical and orthopaedic resident examined the patient, stitched his bleeding wounds, and started medicines. The ward boys and other staff carried the patient to the CT scanner and shifted him to the casualty after the scan. The patient's wife accompanied him throughout. When the senior surgeon came over, the patient requested privacy and revealed that he had recently been diagnosed with HIV and was taking some traditional medicine for that.

At least four college students, the autorickshaw driver, and two ward boys had been exposed to direct contact with his blood. The treating doctors had had their gloves on but not the complete gear expected to be worn while treating such patients (this is usually not made available or compulsory in every casualty). He himself or his wife had not cared to tell the helping hands to protect themselves.

There are umpteen blood-borne diseases, some fatal and many dangerous. While the courts merrily write orders about help for the victim (which is a must), no one cares about the risk to the helper's life while executing such help. No court has ever ordered the government to make universal precaution gear mandatory in hospitals, especially government hospitals where thousands of budding doctors, nurses, ward boys, and technicians are exposed to blood contact daily without knowing the infective status of the patient. It is presumed that the patient is innocent.

Another. A lady of sixty is brought to the casualty unconscious, with a drunk 'mob' led by her son. The son tells that she never had any health problem till that evening, when she had convulsions. They demanded immediate admission in ICU and treatment. The hospital obliged and admitted her as a free patient with an emergency as per court rules. The next morning, the lady revealed that she had had convulsions till a few years ago and was advised regular medicines but had stopped them many days ago. She was also an alcohol addict and had taken alcohol on the prior night. On the day of convulsion, her husband had had a big showdown with her.

Fortunately she went home all well, but one shivers at the idea of what would have ensued had she not improved. Probably another cruelly-beaten-up doctor and voluptuous bad press against the medical fraternity in general.

It is the responsibility of the doctor to be good, perfect, and true in everything he does. But if all the actions and decision-making of this doctor is based upon what the patient tells, any lying or hiding of information by the patient is then likely to impair the outcome. To presume that all patients always tell the truth is a joke.

Many hide addictions. Many hide stigmas—illnesses like tuberculosis, epilepsy, etc. Many hide that they were beaten up by a family member. Many do not tell their drunk status during an accident (many traffic accident deaths, for which the casualty doctors are so often beaten up by relatives, may likely have been avoided had the patient not been drunk).

The most dangerous patients are those who have themselves or because of family pressure neglected the disease until the time it has reached a critical level, often beyond cure. When something happens to such patients in the hospital, our society is quite affected with an innocent media comment: 'The patient was completely all right till admission.'

Some patients do not tell that they missed medicines. Some do not follow precautions. Some take additional herbal, traditional, quackery-born medicines along with the standard treatment without revealing it. The entire responsibility of outcome in every case in any hospital is pinned upon the treating doctor.

While compassion and the art of extracting the correct details are essential for every doctor, it is not mandatory for the patient to tell the complete truth. While repeated questioning may not always be pleasant, it has become necessary to cross-confirm the details for the doctor's own safety and security.

In this medicolegal age in a mostly illiterate, superstitious society, it is essential to educate people about telling the truth and taking precautions while helping others. If you have an open wound, cut, or injury over your own skin, please refrain from touching a bleeding patient. Avoid blood contact with any person unless you are in a position to save a life by taking that risk. It is wise to keep a box of gloves in your car or carry a pair in your purse or office bag for such an emergency where you tend to help.

While it is expected that every doctor, irrespective of how busy he/she is, writes detailed notes and prescriptions in capital letters for every patient, there is no such responsibility assigned to the patient or relative. If the patient is a consumer and the doctor liable for even tiny mistakes or unfavourable outcome, then the clinical/legal responsibility of patients/relatives must also be defined. It must be mandatory for every patient to write the details of their health, prior conditions, all medicines, etc. in legible handwriting and sign it with a witness to submit to the doctor or hospital.

Many patients, educated or not, know this responsibility and carefully and truly detail the doc about everything asked for. They also mostly respect the outcomes. They usually do not blame others or doctor for either their illness or addiction or complications. However, there is a surge nowadays in 'blame it all upon the medic or the hospital'. It is high time some wise judges recognise these issues before deliberating a judgment.

Till then, the medical profession, at least in India, is at the mercy of press interpretation.

CHAPTER 43

THE CURSE OF
REAL HEROES

Two boys, fifteen and eighteen, wheeled in their mom, a spinal case who couldn't walk. They had lost their father guarding the Indian Border. They cared for their mom in turns.

Both wanted to join the army ASAP.

'How much do we pay?' asked the proud elder son after the consult.

'I should pay you with my blood, son!' I wanted to say. But I didn't want to weaken in front of those brave hearts.

'It is my pleasant duty, dear. You don't have to pay,' I told him.

'But this is a private hospital. We can pay. We paid everywhere else we went. We want the best care for our mom.'

'That I promise, and this is in honour of what your father did for all of us.' This made them smile proudly, albeit with a wet twinkle in all eight eyes.

* * *

'I was a Black Cat Commando, sir. I served as a bodyguard to PM Mrs Indira Gandhi, sir,' said this huge, intimidating gentleman, now a victim of Parkinsonism. What an irony that the one known for speed, strength, and accuracy was forced to a life of the opposite! He guarded our prime minister once! He has to go to apply for some medical concession today.

* * *

'I loved this beautiful girl,' said the seventy-five-year-old Punjabi gentleman, pointing at his seventy-two-year-old wife, 'but her father said I was a nobody, so he didn't allow us to marry. Then I won an enemy tank in the war, sent him my picture with it. Then he agreed. I fought three wars for India, sir. But I still cannot dare to fight her, sir.'

You cannot compete with Punjabi humour. He had also been applying the past year to get an accommodation with an elevator facility, as he was on third floor and had to be lifted up by wife and an assistant as he couldn't climb. He had roamed some hospitals in search of relief from a recent illness. He had been admitted at many places and spent a lot of money in this process. He felt it was abuse of the system to claim any concession, as the military hospitals provide adequate healthcare. Naturally, not all patients can be happy with a 'fixed' doctor. They do not have a choice, and if they go to a private hospital, they must pay.

* * *

Young stroke at thirty-two, from Pimpri, Chinchwad. Fighting terrorists in Jammu Kashmir this moment. After recovery from stroke, joined back in anti-terror squad in Assam within four months.

* * *

It is a huge, sticking-out red shame that the very people who endanger their lives for their country without a second thought, who stand in the line of genuine fire, have to live a life of 'requesting, begging, and applying' for favours for basic living: accommodation, transport, food, medicines, and even healthcare of choice, while blatant corruption by many erodes the nation's treasuries.

We live happily at the cost of their risking lives, content with garlanding their memorials twice a year and reposting emotional videos about their sacrifices.

Even the policemen injured while on duty, those who suffered heart attacks, strokes, and other health problems due to an excessively stressful life (the Indian police is almost always overworked) have to stand in line to get memos and recommendation favours from clerical staff to get healthcare concessions. Whatever their alleged level of corruption, it is pathetic to see traffic police at the most polluted junctions standing for the entire day, literally giving away their life.

All healthcare at *any* centre of their choice must be made free for those in the military and policemen who are injured while on duty. Most doctors and private hospitals will agree with this if the medicare-affording patient class that takes advantage of the free facilities is brought to the account book. A rich litany of various political leaders and all their personal staff, ministers and their staff, influential bigwigs, and many undeserving senior government officials take immense advantage of the free and concession system meant for the poor, to investigate and treat themselves, family, and relatives. These unnecessarily 'free' cases number in millions.

There will be some among the military, police who try to take advantage, who may ill-behave, but that can be dealt with if a common health file is maintained for each one, for the doctors to remark so and deny further care in that case.

In a world full of terrorists, the least we can offer as doctors is free treatment to our saviours.

CHAPTER 44

THE SUFFOCATED MEDICAL FUTURE OF INDIA

This simple-looking girl in her early twenties walked into my OPD with her parents. They all were dressed up like the typical lower middle class, just enough to avoid obviously torn clothes. Everything humble, but very well behaved. She started telling her father's complaints in perfect English. As good as a medicine resident doctor would perform in exams, she related the proper history in the correct textbook format, with a polite comment about examination findings. *Excellent case presentation*, I thought.

'Are you a doctor?' My curiosity was awakened by the accuracy of her medical description.

'Yes, sir. I passed out MBBS from BJ, am now doing my compulsory medical officership, then will try for PG.'

A hot knife cut my heart.

She would start PG in her mid-twenties. She will traditionally marry sometime then, have children, and raise a family while slogging as a doctor, while girls her age fully lived their life, proud and rich being a doctor in most of the developed world.

This lady would continue to carry the country's undeserved rural healthcare burden till some arrogant minister, government officer, or local politician

175

got her suspended for not delivering results expected by them, like saving their alcoholic/smoker/aged/chronically diseased/drug-defaulting/multipathy medicating relative admitted at the last moment at midnight after their party was over.

Or else she would keep on begging/applying at multiple corporate set-ups for a decent salary and opportunity, where fresh degree holders from all other non-medical streams who couldn't get enough merit to get into professional courses would make her stand in a queue and ask her for different certificates and proofs of ability, and some perfumed, ill-behaved CEOs would ask her of possible income she could generate and any 'procedural gimmick advantages' she had over others.

Or her teachers would give her sermons on social service being service to God, it being her lifelong duty to serve poor and helpless illiterate patients like they had done, neglecting any of her own desires, especially that of a good life. Or her own richer/well-settled colleagues who earned wealth from prior generations would tell her to 'chill and take things easy'.

Or some court would send her to jail for documentation mistakes. Or peel off her degree as if it was bought undeserved by money.

Or worse, some Bollywood or other celeb with glycerine tears would preach to her how a doctor should be a good human being and never think about money, having chosen this profession.

And like a girl at night in the streets of our country, nobody would protect her.

Among a billion-some population, mostly poor and illiterate, of a disease-ridden country where everyone in government, police, and business continues to get richer by the day, the judiciary body and lawyers take eternity to conclude cases while millions keep on paying both handsomely. The medical fraternity is pushed into hell by all these. PG students are exploited under the 'teaching-learning phase' excuse. They are then posted as medical officers in remote villages as a 'social binding duty' (which lawyers, judges, engineers, ministers, IAS, IPS, and all others can skip) without proper salary (all other classes above have multiple 'helpers' and other benefits). When one emerges from all this compulsory hell, they are left out in the open without any insurance, health or retirement benefits, holidays, loans, etc. Plus a compulsion by law to attend all emergencies they may encounter any time, anywhere, all their lives, with punishment for not attending that emergency.

If the government spends upon the making of a doctor, it is not obliging the doctor, it is doing this for the society whose poverty, illiteracy, and ill health is the government's failure, not the doctor's responsibility. The government should learn to respect the merit of its own best students, extraordinary talents who also have the heart of gold to serve humanity. It should encourage their well-being and provide for their basic needs without pretending to do them a favour. There is nothing more shameful than this: that thousands of 'Made in India' doctors leave the country every year, never to return. Indian doctors practising in other countries earn a name, fame, and wealth far beyond possibilities in India. They are far more productive in clinical, academic, and research areas than those who stay back to tolerate tobacco-chewing, gold-laden, abusive, corrupt freeloader tyrants directly or indirectly in power!

It is a big joke that while most of the doctors slog in rural/backward India to fill up the government's failures with their blood and sweat, the government encourages corporate cultures and business houses in Medicare, and further, accreditation bodies make things glittery so as to earn more! As if the millions of doctors practising in small villages/towns/cities on their own are worthless without such accreditation! Who handles the thousands of epidemics, vaccinations, tubectomies, mother–child care, and emergencies at the rural or grassroots level? Do they have any accreditations? Does any government hospital qualify for any accreditation? Then why has this new accreditation business suddenly cropped up where the patient and doctor are both harassed, while others, including mediclaim (Medical Insurance) companies, earn crores? On top of this, while everyone acts harshly against individual doctors and suspends them at the drop of a hat, the medical bodies are magically and tragically silent about corporate hospitals owned by big business houses, quoting that there are *no rules* against them and medical councils are not authorised to take action against these big set-ups. They can get away with false advertising, harassment of doctors, and even medical negligence without being acted upon by any medical body in India! So anyone with money can form a medical company and start open advertisement about diabetes, heart disease, etc, while the medical bodies are authorised to act only against individuals who do so.

Coming back to the lady doctor in my OPD, I told her that her father may require an MRI. She hesitated for a moment, then her father asked in a shaking voice, 'How much will it cost? We have one thousand rupees only.'

As I begged our kind radiologist for another free MRI (which she granted as always!), I avoided eye contact with the embarrassed family.

If a meritorious young MBBS doctor passing out of a premium government medical college (indicating the highest standards of medical education in India) and working as a medical officer has to beg for basic medical facilities while not being able to properly provide for her own parents, not only us as a profession that has failed to stick together to deserve respect and financial security but also the government, administrative bodies, and medical bodies should all be concerned about this state of affairs of medicine as a profession in India.

CHAPTER 45

THE SILENT, DEADLY MEDICAL BLACKMAIL

A Regular Morning, 10 a.m.

'Do you have the right to say no? I will sue you and the hospital. I will go to the press.' he said humiliatingly.

Very well dressed, from an evidently affluent class, all marks of being highly placed and influential. His father was a highly placed government employee, now in a vegetative state for few months and admitted in another hospital that had the facility to treat government employees under a free scheme. He wanted to shift him to this city. But he wanted his choice of senior doctors to attend his father round the clock. When informed that he could not dictate which consultants should treat the free and government-scheme cases, he threatened as above. He didn't want to pay for any fees/charges for his father's treatment by a team of his choice.

'But my father has served the country for so many years,' he said.

The logical answer would have been 'Have the doctors not been serving the nation too, all their lives? Has your father not raised you and done things for you, made you what you are today, that you are trying to avoid paid medical care for him, fighting for free when you can afford? What is your duty for your father, to avoid all expenses?'

But a doctor must be nice. The doctor gave him the designated team's contact number and explained that hospital policies could not be bypassed.

Also, such patients needed long-term nursing care, and the family often refused to take them home once admitted, thus the availability of hospital beds was then compromised for other deserving patients who needed treatment and could improve.

'This is a shock. We are emotionally shattered by this denial of treatment.'

'Sir, nobody has denied your father any treatment. Only, there are assigned doctors and protocols for this. You need to follow the protocols,' the doctor explained. 'By the way, sir, you must be aware that there are limited beds in any hospital and it is difficult to keep vegetative patients for a long time in such busy hospitals. Other patients, including government and free patients, need admission too, and the beds are already in shortage.'

'I don't care for any of that. Other patients are not my responsibility. My concern is my father. I want the doctors of my choice to treat him as a free case. All doctors only want money. I will complain about this,' said the dutiful son.

'Sir, it is not a question of money. We have unlimited free consultations here. You are welcome to bring in your father any time. Only about admissions, there are protocols.' The doctor was at the end of her patience.

'Now I cannot bring my father as a free patient too because you will hold grudges against him while treating him.'

The doctor lost her patience. You may be very good, but you should never look down upon others. 'You are free to do what you want, sir. We doctors would die every day if we held grudges against everyone who talked ill about doctors. Actually, very few whom we treat respect and talk good about doctors. Even if it is a press reporter, a politician, an actor, or anyone who has blasted, maltreated the doctor, no doctor in the world will treat them with less than her best ability. Of course, we retain the right to deny services to the arrogant, threatening, intimidating, and ill-behaved.' Which other profession has this self-imposed obligation: to do good even unto their enemy? But to explain this is difficult, especially to the money-blinded. He left.

The threatened and insulted doctor called in the next patient from the busy waiting room. She had learnt the act of instantly killing her ego and pushing a smile upon her face after such torturous events, to be ready for the next patient.

* * *

Afternoon, 2 p.m.

This patient needed coiling for an abnormal blood vessel in his brain. Owner of a big private company. Son was a government employee. Five people entered the doctor's room, unfazed by the instruction of only three. Gold shone.

'He must get operated tomorrow. We have admitted him in the general ward, so the operation charge has to be the lowest. We have got the permissions from government offices that he is eligible.'

The accompanying middle-aged khadi-clad 'leader' guy who smelt of alcohol was new. The doctor asked him how he was related to the patient. 'I am like his son,' said the leader.

A look at the clean paperwork confirmed that many a hand had been sweetened for those sanctions. Otherwise, the really deserving poor government employees from lower ranks would keep on knocking doors for even basic tests and medicines.

The coil was not provided by the government or hospital; in such cases, it cost over a hundred thousand rupees sometimes. The doctor informed them so.

'Are you denying treatment?' asked the leader, simultaneously getting up from the chair and adjusting his pants to make the revolver visible. 'I am the leader of XXX party [very notorious reputation] in this city. I hope that you listen and comply, or we have our methods.'

'I am not denying treatment. You will have to talk to the hospital authorities about the coil expenses, as the government does not pay them.'

'We want the patient to be operated tomorrow.'

'Sorry, we cannot book the OT unless everything is arranged in advance.'

In a few hours, the doctor got a call. 'We have arranged for the coil expenses now. He must be operated tomorrow.'

'Please submit the details to the hospital, sir. They will automatically book the OT once formalities are completed,' said the doctor.

The OT was already booked for someone else.

'We don't know. Cancel other bookings,' said the leader.

The expenses, as it became clear, had been made available from a religious charity collecting donations for the poor patient fund.

They got all the free treatment benefit meant for the poor and were happily discharged in a few days. Weeks later, the doctor came to know that there were many such 'leaders' who survived on this business of converting paying patients to free.

* * *

Evening, 9 p.m.

A really poor patient walked in. The old lady had had a stroke and wasn't able to talk or walk; she now came in smiling. Grateful for the free treatment she had received, she wanted to show it. She had learnt a few words. She didn't go to the patient's chair. Instead, she walked to the doctor, pulled the doctor's head down, and caressed her, kissing her forehead, patting the doctor's head. 'I talk now,' she said. She handed over the hundred rupees she had managed to save to gift the doctor, forcing her to accept the note.

This unassuming poor lady had managed to soothe the wounds caused by the powerful blackmailers. The doctor's world was redeemed for that day.

* * *

Night, 3 a.m.

'Ma'am, there's a government employee—a chronic alcoholic with repeated admissions for alcoholic fits—admitted just now, binge-drunk. He had skipped medicines. Vitals now stable. I have loaded antiepileptic. The relatives are drunk too. They want you to see the patient and talk to them. They are creating a ruckus here. They insist that you come immediately.'

The day had started.

CHAPTER 46

WHEN ONCE I MET GOD

Rainy Sunday. My Corolla still young at eight years.

I had just finished rounds and was still irritated at the never-ending task list. From grocery to income tax, there always was something pending, and what was done was never enough. Countless patients with their endless problems, trusting you to solve them, and many suspicious that you have other intentions. Add the cut-throat professional competition where hitting below the belt was a smart move, and frame the picture with the duties towards each relation—the closer, the costlier. Driving through the city, you crossed faceless somebodies flaunting ugly egos. Their middle name was money. Bribe-hungry vampires waited at every corner, dressed in official greed. Nothing to be proud of, nowhere to go, and nobody to look up to.

Life felt like a carcass with vultures on all sides, tearing me away.

Top gear, I entered the expressway and switched on my mental autopilot: the beautiful sound system that was prepared to play the huge collection of music—seventeen thousand tracks, pieces of history encoded in sound, human creation that separated us from animals.

The system burst alive with 'Les Valses de Vienne' by Dmitri Shostakovich/ Francois Feldman, and my brain lit up at the smiling face of my favourite actress, Sophie Marceau, dancing gracefully to the waltz.

Irritability vanished, and a hopeful yearning for good days started whistling to the tune of this eternal piece of music. It hijacks my brain every single time.

183

Born to a shop maid and a truck driver who divorced when she was nine years old, she made to the top in French films and a mark in Hollywood. She must have had her mountains of problems and valleys of a lustful society to overcome before she reached the top, but she indeed made happy memories for the world! It must be so damn difficult to smile and love and dance in front of a camera, knowing this world. Then I felt it: that the beauty is within you—what you can be, what good you do. Nothing outside will ever change, and the mirage of a utopian society will always kick between the legs of most idealists. But at the end of the day, what one will run to, what one will beg for, and what one will regret having lost is this: that all the time one had to do good and feel happy was wasted in feeling bad about what people are and what they do.

The music system, competing with the madness of its owner, shuffled to Simon and Garfunkel's 'El Condor Pasa'. 'A man gets tied up to the ground, | He gives the world its saddest sound.' How tightly we hold on to the ground, never letting go! How religiously we guard the image we like to create of ourselves for others, and how much beauty of life we sacrifice to safeguard that image!

The rain decided to be nice for once and became torrential. If at all it rains, it should rain like the final war, or it should not rain at all!

'Moon River' by Henry Mancini started, as Audrey Hepburn sung in a most loving, melodiously romantic voice what the heart had always craved: 'There's such a lot of world to see | We're after the same rainbow's end.' So many artists have made timeless icons of lovely moments that soak our lives.

God knows how mute love would have been without music, and how dry without the rains!

The uncontrollable desire to get drenched, suppressed for long, took over me. No book said it was unbecoming of a doctor. I parked on the shoulder and got out. Happy raindrops jumped upon my being and got hold of everything I had.

Ironically, the happiest and the saddest moments in life are when you have nowhere to go and nothing to prove. If you hold a hand in the rain, you are the luckiest and richest in the world. If that hand holds your hand with love too, you have lived life.

Steaming hot, poisonously sweet tea made by a roadside vendor added to the flavour of that moment. Like a loving but stern mother slapping upon the bum of her naughty child, nature had shooed human movement, a reminder of the highest rule: enjoy happiness while alive. Big and small, rich and poor, all looked at the sky, content with nothing, smiling at the rain, forgetting the desire to earn more in that moment!

Nostalgic, I recalled sitting by my father and watching water-lily buds broken open by raindrops. I remembered my stunningly beautiful friend with curly hair who kissed me on Marine Drive by the roaring sea under the stormy rain, standing on that parapet, ignoring the shocked people around. I remembered falling flat upon my back like a hundred idiots while running with my kids, just as I was telling them to be careful.

What is it that I am running after now, with so many beautiful things around me: the music, the rain, the friends, my kids, coffee, books, driving, writing . . . What more will I buy that will make these things more meaningful? Is it worth being unhappy, being irritable with the world, trying to change people, having more money than being able to enjoy peacefully?

Once in a recent recorded radio programme, Mr Ameen Sayani, that messiah of voice, played a rare clip of speech by Mr Raj Kapoor: '*Sangeet nahin hota toh jaane hum kahan hote, kya karte, kaise jeete.*' (If there were no music, I wonder where we would be, what we'd do, or how we'd live).

I suddenly realised that the music, the drive, the road, and the rain had conspired to take away my worries. They had reset the method in my madness. The eternal flute, so dearly mentioned in *Gitanjali* by Rabindranath Tagore had played in my heart.

The rain had stopped for now. The music never will.

There, I met God in my own happiness.

CHAPTER 47

QUESTION FROM A YOUNG, FRESH INDIAN DOCTOR

I am pursuing PG after MBBS. I follow your posts regularly. I have a question: Does the passion we harbour to become doctors and serve the society actually fade away? Many of my friends tell me that there's nothing like passion, only money matters after a while, and I should choose a degree that ensures good income. If so, sir, then the corporate culture must be right . . . the more you earn, the better. Then I would be happy to not pursue the PG and start a clinic in villages and be happy with it. Sorry for the long question, but I feel I could get an answer.

Dear next-gen doc,

This answer is going to hurt many within and outside the profession. It will also expect your mature interpretation of what is being said. I beg forgiveness of those who find this unpleasant. In the first part, I will mention some established facts; in the second, I will offer my suggestion to the ever-intelligent younger generation, which is always known to fight and improve upon the situation.

Facts as of now:

1. There is a huge difference in talking about ideal and good and moral and ethical and actually doing it, and unfortunately, we are in a society that blinds itself to this difference. Our society likes people who confidently talk about good and moral, while it harshly punishes/ destroys those who try to unveil truth or hypocrisy. This is why the concept of service to the society is to be carefully interpreted.

2. By saying 'I want to do social service and help the poorest of the poor patients,' we also accept and sanction that this class will always be present in the society. It is a class created by the failures of society and government, not the doctors. If this class was not there (as in if the rural healthcare policies were worked upon and implemented without only the doctors being held responsible for them . . . doctors don't create patients or poverty), most of the Indian population would see a dramatic evolution of better healthcare in India.

3. I do not see many passionate doctors now. Most who started out with the golden dream of living a respected, settled life and social gratitude for serving humanity are frustrated coping up with their rents, children's school fees, midsize car loans, restrictions, and new rules by governments that leave the rich and powerful and corporates out but shred the careers and lives of individual/small/middle-class medical practitioners.

4. The society or the government does not care if a doctor who has served it all his life dies of poverty, sickness, accident, occupational risk, etc. There is no example of a good doctor's family having been helped by society after his death. There is no insurance or protection or retirement benefit in return of medical social service of a doctor.

5. If it were only a question of serving and earning respect, let me tell you that patients make their own choices always, and there is nothing wrong in that. But they will seldom stand by you in case of any mistake/problem you face, beyond curiosity and sympathy. On top of this, you are at the wish and whim of different laws, rules, regulations,

etc. made by those who neither studied medicine nor practised it, especially in villages. They can call, humiliate, dictate, transfer, ask for a bribe, disrespect, or ask personal favours from you, and still treat you like a servant, irrespective of whether you have done Nobel Prize–worthy social service.

6. A culture of choosing high-earning postgraduate degrees has been encouraged in India, a nation of perpetually low-income intellectuals, who often have to avail of loans for education and grow up with the natural desire of living a good, respectable, and comfortable life, like everyone else. The government, parents, teachers, senior doctors, etc.—everyone has silently witnessed this process over years. However, we also have a highly pseudo-moral society, which expects service and honesty at the cost of a doctor's life without providing for his needs according to his socio-intellectual standing, hard work, and skill. So whatever your education may be in the medical field, if you follow all the laws and criteria of patient satisfaction, the equation is pretty screwed up: that you cannot see more than twenty patients in a day; you cannot advertise as an individual and so have no way to compete with hospitals or sophisticated quacks who can advertise as they wish. The ethics and morals that individuals must follow do not apply to hospitals.

There are umpteen impractical restrictions by government or some other bodies, even upon the most critical surgeries/procedures. This restricts the income way too much, thus encouraging malpractice. Lower-income PG seats are the last choice, and the PGs that have procedures/surgeries have become a preferred choice because of multimodal incomes in these. Naturally, medical care is becoming more invasive. Also, the awareness of the educated about medical procedures makes things worse, as they think that the best must also come cheapest.

7. Medical success is measured by many a desperate doctor as medallions from the government, money, and big hospital buildings, and the social and media image of a godman or messiah. They have the money (how? does not matter) and they have the fame (for being present longest in the field from a time there was no competition or even

rules), so they go on advising moral and ethical floral bouquets to the younger generation docs publicly but aim at pleasing the media and the low-intellect masses that highly depend upon the media to form their opinion. I would like to know how many 'rich and famous' doctors from earlier generations have helped needy younger-generation doctors with money/scholarships for higher education. Most PG seats have been created to earn more by selling degrees.

In a country that boasts of some of the best doctors in the world, how many researchers in any field have won a Nobel Prize?

May I please make a suggestion?

Never underestimate your passion. It is the most important thing in life to pursue. But first, know your correct passion/calling without thinking of something to impress others. You should be able to live with it irrespective of what people say about it, and you should be able to accept perpetual failure for that one passion—then alone does it qualify as your true passion. Finances, fame, and social acceptance are not the aims of any passion.

The decision to live a life of low income is not easy and is to be made only with the consent of your dependents/family; they did not sacrifice their active life so that you wouldn't take care of them in their needy times. Your duty to take good care of your parents and children cannot be neglected. You may choose to pursue your passion without compromising upon these responsibilities. You will have a husband or wife and kids to raise, and it would be a great injustice to your kids if you don't provide them with a good and healthy childhood and education. Which Indian village has this? Also, for a good married life, you need to spend time with your spouse; otherwise, you are doing him/her injustice. So if you have to do social service, first obtain a consent for this decision from your family, beloved, and dependents.

If your passion is for medicine, do not combine it with social service. Get your degree, go for higher education or research (both of which are pathetically lagging at least fifteen years behind the developed world, and no one seems ashamed of this) and make yourself proud by working in a developed country that does justice to your medical talent.

If your passion is to medically serve the Indian poor patients, do not expect any financial remuneration, recognition, or respect. I will personally respect you as a form of God, like the thousands who are actually doing this right now, all over India, without any recognition. Some of these are in government service, some are individual, and some are hospital practitioners. A few with good connections get prizes, medallions, recognitions, etc., and most of them are at either fag end of their career. But then be prepared like myself to have to apply for loans, beg financial favours from people who will advise you about career, and take advantage of you every which way they can.

I had made a conscious choice to return to India after the highest education as a passion towards serving the poorest of the poor, and I have been made to regret this choice by a silent earlier generation of practitioners who didn't care what happened to next generation; an inert government that really does not care about public health, patients, or doctors in general; a corporate culture that works purely as a profit-making business; impractical rules/regulations not contested by medical bodies; and a society that prefers not to look beyond immediate selfish motives.

There is hope; I am optimistic still (that's why I am still writing this, staying here). But we now need a medical revolution.

I absolutely do not mean any disrespect towards the senior generation, including my teachers, who made me what I am today. I only mean that most of those who were in a position and power to make changes did not do so. I have seen and witnessed closely the financial and social (sometimes legal) frustration of many teachers who had abilities par excellence and skills of a world-class doctor but had to live perpetually in a state of financial insecurities. In spite of this, they have always encouraged ethical and moral behaviour from us students.

I must mention at the same time that if I give impractical advice, which will push my students into a life of desperation, frustration, and dependence, I will feel guilty about it.

Make a wise decision, and may God bless you.

CHAPTER 48

MILORD, PLEASE DON'T TRY THIS MEDICINE!

An old saying 'The young man knows the rules, but the old man knows the exceptions' seems to keep our judicial officers forever young. The following article is not for a comparison between doctors and legal professionals (my best friend is a lawyer, and I owe many a reasoning skill and tea bill to him).

Not always while learning medicine could we understand or agree with some decisions made by our seniors, as they either contrasted with the 'textbook' instructions or were never mentioned anywhere; it was the sheer genius and practical experience of those seniors that often saved lives. Such risks were almost always well calculated against the risk of death and discussed with patient's relatives whenever they had a capacity to understand (rare). We have never seen a doctor working/acting with the intention of 'causing harm' to the patient.

There are often (not at all rare) situations when even two of the world's best authorities do not agree upon some medical issue. This is beyond most of the 'average IQ' people to comprehend, those who can only understand the most simplified. It is not because of a clash of egos but a tie between two dead ends.

This is why medical definitions and management guidelines change very frequently. This is why every practising doctor becomes a criminal by law, having 'bypassed' some guideline somewhere in his/her career for doing good to the patient who did not fit in the medical definition or was not mentioned in the textbooks.

It takes about six years to become a basic allopathic doctor and about fifteen years to become a medical specialist. Only half of this training is in the books; the remaining half is the actual experience of dealing with the thousands of complicated medical problems and learning to untangle the situation by extremely difficult decision-making. But we see some specialists do very well as compared to others, and to presume it is only because they 'cut practice' is intellectual poverty! Most doctors who do well do so because of their exceptional abilities in their field, especially in this society with such a bias against doctors as a class!

Legal training does not include medical knowledge and reasoning; it usually deals with other crimes like rapes, thefts, financial- and property-related crimes, sexual aberrances, poisonings, murders etc. Beyond that, a lawyer would have to make a special effort to learn from prior judgments about the precedents set mostly in the Western world. To apply these directly to the Indian medical practice is impractical and humorous. We have a legal system that has many differences from the Western system: be it relationships, marriages, sex, rapes, political crimes, or homosexuality. In most of these, the judges quote Indian culture and the difference in society. Separate laws and courts have evolved where industries and money was concerned. Military conducts its own trials/courts martial.

But the most intellectually complicated field dealing with human life is left out to be handled by people who may be very good in law but have little or no knowledge of the intricacies involved in handling a complicated medical case. Most of the judges and lawyers, with due respect, would lack the basic knowledge about the unpredictability of various medical treatments, procedures, and clinical outcomes, despite the best medical brains involved in these cases.

Summarily, doctors in general are as law-dumb as those not doctors are medical-dumb. To allow anyone except medical professionals to either make laws or to try doctors in courts that have had no medical training or acumen (which, incidentally, takes years of day and night training in hospitals) is like asking an MBBS doctor to analyse and criticise the decisions of a Supreme Court judge. We are so mentally enslaved to the ancient British system that we have to rise and salute the authority of every judge because they are so 'highly placed'—socially, legally, and ethically, that a doctor who deals with human life, who saves hundreds in his lifetime, has to beg them with folded hands. Beg them to understand that he/she was trying to save a human life, and they decide the merit based upon their puny medical knowledge, which is unchallengeable!

Some laws practised today were made over one hundred years ago. Medical science changes daily. Only the sane and solid minds will sense the paradox here. We need separate medical courts. Thousands dying due to incorrect political decisions and accidents do not receive even pebbles as compensation despite knocking the doors of all courts, but a single inadvertent medical mistake is punished with multimillion rupees' compensation, a lifetime income beyond 95 per cent doctors in our country!

Yes. Doctors should not have to stand in regular courts begging mercy for trying to do good. They must have medical courts with special judges who have adequate (at least MBBS level) knowledge about the human body and are also trained in it as well in law. Only a multidisciplinary panel of young and old doctors and legal experts can properly analyse the merits or otherwise of a medical case. Or the medical council should conduct qualifying examinations for judges who conduct medicolegal cases or train them with experts from various super specialties about the basic principles of a doctor's approach to complicated medical issues. They must also be aware about the non-medical issues that kill a patient (delay in admission, addictions, health neglect, non-compliance with advised tests/treatment, neglect by family, etc.), which never appear in legal discussions of negligence cases.

I have immense respect for the judiciary and its abilities; I have immense faith in its intentions. However, being a doctor, I cannot harbour superstitions or blind faith. I *do not* believe that the regular judges or doctors will understand all that happens in a spaceship travelling to Mars; only the astronauts can understand those intricacies. I do not believe that anyone who has not composed the same music as Mozart or Tchaikovsky or A. R. Rahman or Ilayaraja should criticise them.

The present tradition of any court trying medical cases can only be equated to the legal system punishing an acclaimed singer for singing a wrong note! Unfortunately, as this profession concerns life, the 'wrong note' or *bigda sur* can result in health complications. But then to completely avoid it, one must stop singing.

This is also why most good new-generation Indian doctors are leaving India. Not that there are better judges outside but there are better payments for the frustration involved!

If not anything else, my dear and most respectable milord, sir, please understand the dire necessity of a duress-free doctor the society deserves.

CHAPTER 49

THE BEAUTY
CALLED BRAIN

I can't ever adequately express the beauty of the neuronal organisation within the brain. I keep realising again and again that it feels far more rewarding to study than to explain it, to understand its poetic yet mathematically perfect logic rather than to describe the names of its components, to know that it functions as beautifully without one's even being aware of it, to be amazed of its abilities which surpass our capacities to grasp them, and to know that they have kept us alive and going before we could think or be aware of our own existence, before we knew any language!

The language that the brain uses is more beautiful than any known, however ancient, that can form a bond between animals and humans, between animals of different species, the language of compassion, of natural discipline of not killing except for hunger and self-protection, the language that newborns speak through their touch with their mother, or the meeting of eyes that communicate terabytes of feelings in a glance, the ultra-beautiful feeling of falling in love when you meet the right person, the gift of understanding without having spoken a word!

While the abilities of our brains far exceed our ability to understand them, the simple fact that everything in the cosmos can be compared with, can be expressed within a human brain itself, declares the vastness of this 'gateway to the universe' that probably has the solutions for achieving world peace; ending hunger and wars, crime and violence; discovering eternal happiness and maybe even attainment of perpetual bliss for every single soul during life, but we humans have chosen to use it instead for monies, religions, power, property, sex, fame, and satisfaction of ego by defeating, showing down, and making slaves of people under different sweet titles.

We, inferior to our own brain, try to enslave this master, forcing it to learn and repeat and train itself into doing mundane things. Just because the master is kind enough to allow us complete freedom to choose what we do with it.

The song that every brain naturally sings is the mother hymn of all humanity, if only we could listen to it silently!

If anyone has the capacity to redeem us from the material mess humanity has collectively created, it is the human brain, used correctly.

Wishing so desperately.

CHAPTER 50

BEWARE OF THIS DREADFUL DISEASE

'Why isn't she improving, Doc?' asked the eager chartered accountant. His wife had been visiting many specialists for headaches, sleep trouble, and tiredness. 'She is also putting on weight because of the medicines so many doctors have given her.'

His wife, in her early thirties, sat there, tearful, and stared angrily at the table between us. Their kids were at home with his parents. They had returned from the United States to settle in India, and she had a small job too at an art gallery.

* * *

'Why?' The same question—this time the wife had recurrent episodes of unconsciousness. All tests normal. The husband was a political leader of the B type, with an intimidating and heavy bodybuilder personality. The couple had tonnes of gold upon them.

'We have everything. She does not have to move even a finger at home. We have many servants. But she keeps on crying without a reason. I think she has psychological problem,' said Goldy the bodybuilder.

His wife sobbed throughout the consult without speaking a word.

* * *

'What exactly is the problem?' asked this Indian Londoner who brought her father for forgetfulness. She visited him regularly, once a year. Her brother who stayed in India had chosen not to meet parents, being busy with his wife and kids. The old man stayed here with his paralysed wife. His children had split the monies and the hearts.

'I make sure that we send them enough money for a good-quality life,' said the daughter. 'We have hired them a home in a senior locality, where he can make friends. They also have a visiting doctor and physiotherapist. But Papa does not make friends with anyone, and his weight is also reducing now. He seems lost all the time.'

* * *

'Who is the best doctor for such cases in the world?'

Twelve-year-old girl with recent episodes of abnormal behaviour. Parents both high-profile professionals: father mostly travelling, mother in office all day. Now there was no babysitter as the kid had grown up, she was very intelligent; and used to get good marks in school till the previous year.

'I can take her to any doctor anywhere in the world if you suggest,' said the father. 'Tell us the best specialist in the world. I want the correct diagnosis and treatment as fast as possible.'

* * *

The name of the disease in all these cases: Lacklove Syndrome.

Here, the ones who asked the questions were the patients. They failed to understand that the people who depended upon them for gentle, loving care, empathy, and interaction were suffering because these 'lackloves' thought that money, gold, or facilities would replace the most basic human need: love.

Thousands of families suppress the individuality of their own dependents, force upon them customs and traditions which they themselves do not follow. Cute names to the relationship and pretension of caring are false masks hiding the true face of a New Age devil—material, loveless relationships.

There is a life-and-death difference between actually loving and talking about love. Even animals understand the difference; we humans pretend to mask it with too many words and material proofs. True love between two living beings precludes both: words or proofs.

The other side: marrying for money or status, choosing life-options entirely driven by material gains, investing only in the 'earning virtues' of children are also the guarantees of an unpleasant future. Not knowing the life partner and their life preferences is a big gamble in an educated, hence wiser, world.

In the first case, the wife was an artist and revealed later that it was impossible for her to 'connect' to her husband, who was not interested in art or conversation and didn't enjoy anything beyond his finance-related work.

In the second case, the wife's sister had recently died of cancer at an early age, and she required someone to reassure and be tender to her. Goldy the bodybuilder was never trained for that.

The old father, in the third case, wanted to be with his children in these last years. 'That was my dream,' he said.

The child in the last case was too scared to be alone at home and had no one to talk to. 'Once, I just told about bullying at school to my father, but he came to the school and blasted my principal. So my teachers are angry with me now,' the kid said.

We desperately need love and art training in our schools, along with science, languages, and maths.

CHAPTER 51

A MODERN DOCTOR'S CURSE: SISYPHEAN OLD-AGE OATHS AND ETHICS

What a paradox that in science, where almost every textbook mentions on the first page that 'medicine is an ever-changing science', we lack a social, medical, and ethical philosophy that can ensure medical care without exploitation of a doctor!

The importance of the Hippocratic Oath is beyond any disrespect, and its status of being Document 1 in the medical sciences will remain undisputed. But if anyone in today's world presumes and expects a BC-dated principle to apply uniformly all over a world full of social, constitutional, political, cultural, economic, sexual, legal, genetic, and religious differences, they are either intellectually challenged or reality perverts.

There are many improvisations on many different oaths till now. However, one cannot apply a principle globally without prior globalization of the science/ art/religion to which such a principle is being applied.

So then, what a doctor is expected to follow all over the world, the governments, the paramedical set-ups, the insurance companies, and even the patients are expected to fall in line with. Do they?

Would Hippocrates have accepted today that the insurance companies decide what the doctors should do and what they charge? That the governments do not pay doctors well, that the ministers and judges and all sorts of rich and powerful actually take advantage of a system they govern and consider their own health and life *above* others? That there are rules for individual practitioners but not medical institutes? That the doctors suffer overwork, stress, and underpayment in most societies based upon unidirectional ethics? That patients, relatives, politicians, and police beat up and sometimes kill doctors who were trying to save lives?

Much of our society and media (which reminds doctors of their oaths regularly) is like the playboy husband who enforces upon his wife the cultural and traditional principles of extreme loyalty, obedience, and dedication to him and family while he himself jumps over the moral fence often.

The point is not justification of what is unethical, immoral, or corrupt— that is ruled out as incorrect—it is about impractical and illogical expectations.

Good has to be created in wakefulness by reforms, not only dreamt in sleep.

The old-age oaths and ethics professors never considered the following factors:

1. corrupt governments enforcing wrong/incomplete healthcare policies, binding upon the doctors

2. doctors' councils sanctioning licenses to the corrupt for bestowing degrees without merit or proper eligibility, also allowing doctors to cross doctrines.

3. Mediclaim/insurance companies operating as profit-making businesses, governing and curtailing the remunerations of a doctor.

4. governments entirely dumping their responsibilities towards the health of all the poor only upon the doctors without providing any backup, facilities, or remuneration.

5. the discrepancy in population explosion in the face of an always limited number of doctors, overworked all over the world.

6. the legal system formed by those who did not study the extremely complicated science of medicine presuming it will correctly interpret it and trying to decide and punish the doctors

7. the patients/society in general spending upon all other luxuries but not considering health as a necessary expense.

8. Do No Harm not applying to both sides (No oath or ethic can say that the doctor should let suffer his health, joy, family ties, and a good life)

9. 'Medical shopping' by many patients—this itself tells of difference in the quality of doctors and hence rules out any 'capping'. If capping of charges is implemented, the doctors should refuse second/third opinions because that will be against the principle of equality then!

It is left only to the medical practitioner to be innocent, ethical, and selfless; he must shut up and serve under the name of an oath made by a great soul more than two thousand years ago!

The whole scenario of medical science in the age of Hippocrates may have been considered as a limited facility where only the patient (presumably straight, innocent, religious, and ethical) and the doctor were involved.

If ethics worked in only one direction, the best example to compare is imagining Mahatma Gandhi in a city of today's hardcore criminals and terrorists.

Institutions that employ doctors, governments that fail while those in power get rich, and most diagnostic facilities, pharmaceuticals, and medical insurance companies all work openly for making profits (This includes most in the society too!), so the doctor, who is the only face of all these for the patient, bears the brunt of patient's anger. None of the above bodies is controlled by the doctors!

It is utterly stupid if people expect that the most talented and hardworking will always voluntarily sacrifice their lives and pleasures for a society that thinks of medical service as a one-way ethical path. Most doctors have worked hard and also want to practise ethically, but if that contrasts with their own health, happiness, peace of mind, and family, they will quit for a better country, career, or choice.

The new mindset should be 'I will pay for my best health, and if I want a good, non-corrupt doctor, I will understand that his/her fees will be more than those who malpractice.' Patients who look for 'cheap' everywhere, may risk endangering their lives, as there are many malpractices either neglected or sanctioned by the governments. The maximum duping of patients happens not by the doctor but by most other medical and non-medical profit makers involved in healthcare.

May I suggest the following:

The doctor should do no harm to any patient, and patients also should do no harm to any doctors.

The doctor should behave best with the patient; the patient should also behave best with the doctor. Trust and understanding should be bilateral.

The doctor should work in the best interest of the society, and society should also work in the best interest of its doctors.

The doctor should respect the patient's privacy and do best for his/her patient according to the his/her ability, and the patient must also have complete faith and trust in the doctor's ability and intention to do so. Then there is no question of legal action. In case of proven negligence, the same charges that were to be paid by the patient had the outcome been good must be the amount of punishment paid by the guilty doctor.

The doctor should forgive the patient's mistakes (addictions, wrong history, lies, hidden information, lost records, neglect of their own health, bad behaviour, request for illegal/false documentation or certifications, etc., which the doctor cannot comply with, and also the daily risk to the doctor's life), and the patient will also forgive the doctor's mistakes.

A doctor should not accept or contribute to any corruption, and anyone concerned with the health services—government, pharmaceuticals, medical councils, Mediclaim companies, and patients themselves—should also not accept or contribute to any corruption, unethical practices, excessive profit-making, etc.

Patients/relatives who provide wrong/false/incomplete/manipulated information to the doctor and who threaten or pressurise the doctor should be as liable for legal action as a doctor committing a mistake, because all these factors seriously affect healthcare by endangering the patient's life and wasting the doctor's precious time.

For every free or concessional patient that a doctor is supposed to treat, there should be an income tax benefit equal to the amount of that treatment. There should also be exemption from income tax for a doctor's and his family's retirement benefits equivalent to an upper-middle-class salary. This is the minimum expectation from doctors, whom the society expects to serve themselves at all times.

Unless the society ensures good life and peace of mind for the doctors, which comes with proper remunerations, security, and freedom to make the best decisions for patients without legal, social, criminal, political duress, the healthcare systems will remain critically ill and upon the verge of crisis.

CHAPTER 52

THE BEST MOMENTS IN A DOCTOR'S LIFE

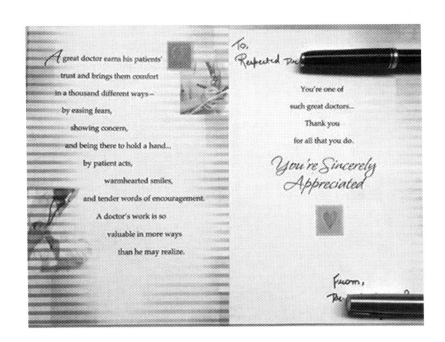

1. The sound of restarting heartbeats when resuscitating a patient.

2. Closure after a difficult surgery, where only the surgeon knows how he/she has saved a life.

3. A perfect surgery or procedure, coiling or stenting without complication.

4. Seeing the beautiful, cute face of a healthy newborn.

5. Managing a major bleeder successfully.

6. Reversal of paralysis after thrombolysis (clot-buster injection).

7. Termination of status epilepticus (non-stop seizures/convulsions).

8. Control over infection. Every infection is life-threatening potentially.

9. Waking up of a comatose patient.

10. The genuine 'Thank you' of a patient relieved of pain/stress/illness.

11. When someone random recognises you in public and thanks you in front of your kids/family.

12. When the poorest of the poor collect enough money and gift you something as a token of gratitude for free treatment.

13. When a patient too educated to believe your truth goes to your professional competitors and many others and is told the same so returns to you with a greater faith.

14. When you can answer all questions asked by students after a lecture/ clinic (without bluffing).

15. When your students perform well and the patients give you good feedback about them.

16. When you silently prove your clinical argument with good results.

17. When anyone at work says, 'Take some rest now. You have been working too much.'

18. Qualifying for a medal, degree, or publication of significant repute.

19. When you know that it's not only the medical skills but also your passionate involvement, speed, and coordination that saved the patient.

20. When traffic police let you go for minor offences just because you are a doctor, especially on the way to an emergency.

21. When someone says, 'I want to become a doctor like you'.

There are many more. Every day is filled with both tears and smiles, and the doctor has to balance these by using his/her soul as the fulcrum. At the end of the day, death humbles everyone, but it is the doctor who stands to defend everyone else's life without thinking if they are good or bad, friend or enemy.

Who will believe that money, home, family, cars, looks, luxury, and even love and romance are secondary joys for most doctors after they have attended all their patients' issues?

This pride is precious. The suffering is a choice. The rewards . . . who cares? A good doctor is the best a human being can be.

Printed in the United States
By Bookmasters